THE
FINAL HURDLE

A Physician's Guide to Negotiating a Fair Employment Agreement

DENNIS HURSH, ESQ.

Copyright © 2019, 2012 by Dennis Hursh

This publication is designed to provide accurate and authoritative information in regard to the subject matter covered. It is sold with the understanding that the publisher is not engaged in rendering legal, accounting, or other professional services. If legal advice or other expert assistance is required, the services of a competent professional person should be sought.

Dedication

My first-born daughter was born with DiGeorge Syndrome, complicated by a rare, complex heart defect. This book is dedicated to the residents, fellows and attendings who worked tirelessly over endless days and nights as she endured six open heart surgeries, thousands of seizures, a spinal fusion and a bout with bacterial endocarditis that nearly took her life.

I have dedicated my career to helping physicians like them navigate the world of employment contracts so that they can focus on doing what they do best – healing the sick and injured.

It is a small repayment of a personal debt that can never be fully repaid – my beautiful, healthy daughter is now 29 years old, and happily living life on her own special terms. This could not have happened without the hard work of countless physicians, and it is my goal to increase physician career satisfaction in whatever way I can.

Thanks can never be enough.

About the Author

Dennis Hursh, Esq., has been a practicing attorney since 1982. He has focused on representing physicians in contractual matters since 1992, when he founded Hursh & Hursh, P.C. His legal peers in the healthcare law field have rated him AV ("preeminent").

After graduating from Dickinson College in 1976 and then Penn State Dickinson School of Law in 1982, Hursh received his master's degree in the laws of taxation from Georgetown University Law Center in 1985. He also served as both an active-duty and reserve Marine Corps infantry officer for more than twenty years.

Hursh, a frequent lecturer at residency and fellowship programs, has spoken at events sponsored by the Pennsylvania Medical Society, the Penn State Milton S. Hershey Medical Center, the Pinnacle Health System, the Geisinger Health System, the Pennsylvania Society of Cardiology, the WellSpan Health System, the Hospital of the University of Pennsylvania, and the American Podiatry Association.

Hursh also founded the Physician Prosperity Program®, the nation's premier contract review and negotiation service. The Physician Prosperity Program® provides comprehensive compensation analysis utilizing nationally recognized benchmarks, as well as detailed legal review of physician employment agreements. An experienced physicians' contract attorney will also negotiate the final agreement, if desired.

Hursh and his wife, Yvonne, have four children: Rachel, John, Lydia, and Ben. He is an active in member at the Unitarian Church of Harrisburg and enjoys trips to the range with his children (although he admits that his days of qualifying as a Marine Corps expert marksman are long past). He has also served as co-chair of the Patient and Family-Centered Care Advisory Council of the Penn State Milton S. Hershey Medical Center and as co-chair of the Penn State Hershey Children's Hospital's Family Advisory Council.

He is an actively practicing attorney in Pennsylvania, whose practice is focused on the review of physician employment agreements in all 50 states.

Hursh can be reached by telephone at (866) DOC-LAW1 or at (717) 930-0600. He also can be reached by e-mail at Dennis@PaHealthLaw.com. For information about the Physician Prosperity Program®, please visit www.PaHealthLaw.com.

Table of Contents

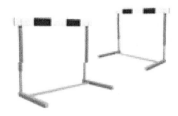

Introduction: Stars in Your Eyes

Imagine that you have completed all your courses and passed all your exams, and are finally ready to take your first position. You have diligently pursued every lead, and now you have impressed the individual who does the hiring at a workplace you feel would be a good fit.

The physician-in-charge has taken you out to the nicest restaurant in town (your spouse, if you had time for a social life at some point in your educational career, may have come too). The food is superb and fine wine is flowing. You and the physician are having an animated discussion. You feel this person really understands the sacrifices you have made and already views you as a worthy colleague.

The candlelight, great food, and interesting conversation (and, perhaps, the wine) are giving you a sense of collegiality and belonging. This job is starting to look like

1

a lock! You are already savoring the offer that is virtually certain to come along. You feel that those monstrous student loans really can be paid off and you will still be able to live comfortably, almost luxuriously. It all just feels right.

The physician you are chatting with leans toward you and says, "You seem like a perfect fit! We'll send you our standard contract, which we all have signed. Of course, like the rest of us, you'll be agreeing not to practice medicine in this city if for some reason you ever leave us. You don't have any problem with that, right?"

This seems like a no-brainer. "Of course not!" you hurriedly exclaim. It's a great salary with great people, and everybody else has agreed to it, so why on earth wouldn't you agree too?

Whoa there, Doc!

It is perfectly natural for you to want to show you are a team player at this point. After all, you have worked your butt off to get where you are. You have excelled throughout your academic career and through all the hard years of your residency (and maybe through a fellowship, too). Your compensation to this point has been slightly above subsistence – probably not as much as you would have been paid if you had worked at minimum wage for all those hours of studying, working, teaching, and covering call. If you are in a committed relationship, your significant other has endured a great deal to support you up to this point. Your educational loans are likely in the hundreds of thousands of dollars; you may feel that you are drowning in debt.

Instinctively grabbing for the first life preserver offered is only natural.

Still, at this point you desperately need both practical advice and expert guidance as you deal with the process of obtaining your first position. The simple fact is that the world of academic medicine is somewhat insular. Nobody would question your keen intelligence and you have obtained, through plain hard work, an incredible amount of highly specialized knowledge. However, analyzing compensation structures and contractual terms for physician employment agreements is another "specialty" altogether. Just when you thought the race was over, you're suddenly looking at an unexpected final hurdle. You can't stumble now! You need a consult – stat!

 So, even though you're a trained specialist, analyzing the complexities of a physician employment agreement is another specialty altogether. Just when you thought the race was over, you're suddenly looking at an unexpected final hurdle. You can't stumble now! You need a consult – stat!

You have sobering responsibilities, both to yourself and to those you love, and you must make the best possible decisions at this critical juncture. The first contract you accept will influence the rest of your life, not just your professional career. It is vitally important to use every

3

resource available to you to assure the best possible outcome.

At times in this book, I advise you to play the "dumb doc." Please don't be offended – this charade is simply a negotiation tactic that can be handy in several circumstances. You can gain time to consider a proposition, for example, or you can say it's your advisers, not you, who are critical of the offer. By explaining with a smile that you "really don't understand this legal and business stuff," you can take full advantage of your advisers' expertise. By the way, you are likely to see this tactic used against you at least once during recruitment and negotiation, so just recognize the tactic for what it is and go with the flow.

In this book, I will tell you about the critical elements in every physician employment agreement, whether you are employed by a hospital, a private practice, or the government. Although each offer will be different, these critical elements should always be addressed. The following paragraphs constitute a sampling of what you will learn.

COMPENSATION

The first element you need to look at is the compensation offer. You've worked hard to get where you are and those huge medical school debts aren't going to pay themselves. The starting compensation in your first contract is likely to be the basis of all future increases – so you need to make sure your initial compensation is appropriate.

In this book, you'll learn how to assess the offered compensation accurately, find out what benchmarks are available, and discover what the limitations of those benchmarks are. We will also discuss gauging the productivity level an employer is likely to expect for a given compensation amount. You'll gain a basic understanding of some common methods of compensation determination and some pitfalls inherent in those methods.

Of course, your compensation package will be much more than just a salary. We'll also talk about your likely benefits package, which includes some of the other important benefits (CME, board certification and recertification fees, vacation, medical staff dues, and so forth) that should also be offered.

RESTRICTIVE COVENANTS

You'll also discover the shocking consequences that restrictive covenants could have for your career. A restrictive covenant is a binding agreement to restrict your medical activities when you leave an employer. Too many physicians take their prospective employer's word for how (un)important a restrictive covenant's provisions are, or they mistakenly believe those provisions cannot be enforced.

A restrictive covenant's two major components are the area it covers and the restriction's time period. These provisions hold numerous traps for the unwary. We'll discuss the major elements you need to analyze in order to determine whether a restrictive covenant is reasonable.

PERFORMANCE REQUIREMENTS

We'll also delve into key requirements of your anticipated position as set forth in the employment contract. Many initial offers have language about call coverage that is so vague that the employer can assign 24/7 coverage without violating the agreement. While the employer's size will tend to determine how specific call coverage requirements are, you can often get some general assurances to protect you from getting more than your fair share of call. I'll give you guidance for evaluating the language in these provisions and what is reasonable. (I probably won't be able to tell you how to avoid being on call on Christmas your first year, though).

Your first employment contract should include general productivity and working-hour provisions. The agreement should have reasonable requirements for patient contact hours. Remember that charting doesn't end when you get out of training – 40 hours of patient contact equates to a lot more than 40 hours of work.

You will learn about the provisions concerning when employment starts. You'll also learn about pitfalls: a physician might move to a new location in anticipation of a new position, only to be refused the right to begin earning a salary until meeting conditions that are out of his or her control. We will also discuss the extremely critical provisions that govern how you and the employer can terminate the employment relationship.

I've seen agreements requiring the physician to respond to all e-mails within two hours – presumably, for 24 hours a day. We'll talk about some of the common provisions you might encounter and which ones could be a big problem for you.

MALPRACTICE INSURANCE

You'll learn the vital facts about malpractice insurance. In general, there are two types of coverage: "occurrence" and "claims-made." There is little difference between these types of coverage while you are with the employer. However, there is a huge difference between them after you leave a given employer. Claims-made insurance will no longer cover you for alleged acts or omissions during your employment, and "tail coverage," which covers this gap, can cost as much as a third of a year's salary. You'll learn how to protect yourself so you never get stuck in a situation where the cost of getting out and purchasing your own tail coverage is prohibitive.

OWNERSHIP

Many physicians will accept a position with a private practice. If this applies to you, you'll want to know how and when you'll become an owner. We'll talk about what the first employment agreement should include regarding eventual ownership and what you probably shouldn't expect. One of the provisions your first employment contract with a private practice should include is determining a buy-in's purchase price, if you are offered ownership.

There are many ways of determining the purchase price for buying into a private practice. This determination is generally based on one of three methods:

1. Par value of the underlying security (e.g., stock in a professional corporation, partnership interest in a limited liability company, etc.) or some other fixed dollar amount. This method may produce a cheap buy-in price, but that may not be in your best interest, for reasons I'll discuss later.
2. Fair market value. This method may seem "fair", but it is likely to lead to a great deal of friction between you and the practice when the time comes to buy in and figure out the price.
3. Book value. This method will use some variation of the value of the practice's assets, as reflected on the practice's books, to arrive at the purchase price of your buy-in. This can lead to an expensive buy-in: we'll talk about some of the advantages of this method, as well as issues that may arise from it.

RECRUITMENT AGREEMENTS

We'll discuss some of the key issues that present themselves if a health system is involved in recruiting you to work at a private practice. You'll learn why I try to limit the repayment periods in these agreements, and why these agreements may allow you to increase the compensation or benefits offered while the practice is using "other people's money." We will talk about strategies to generally avoid personal liability for any repayment requirement, and also tax considerations that should be factored into the agreements.

NEGOTIATION STRATEGIES

We'll also talk about the best negotiation strategies to use throughout this process. Above all, I want you to understand that negotiations begin with the first recruitment call. Too many doctors give away the farm before the first offer is even produced.

You must not be passive and pliant about negotiations. Your prospective employer is likely to conclude that you just don't care very much about contract provisions that are naturally important to that employer. Once that conclusion is made, your chances of getting a reasonable offer are greatly diminished. You must be firm, yet amicable; it can be difficult to find just the right balance.

I've been reviewing and negotiating physician employment agreements since 1992, and I've seen some provisions that were truly atrocious, even with the benefit of all those years of negotiations. Generally, the attorneys involved truly care about getting the best deal possible for their clients, with results that are a win for each party. The benefit of these workarounds can be used in future negotiations, as the attorney becomes adept at discerning which variations work for both parties. Every physician employment agreement an experienced attorney works on tends to be better than the one before.

The secret all experienced attorneys know is that every contract is negotiable. I have obtained concessions on important provisions from both massive health systems and small private practices. When the person you are dealing with tells you that you have been given the "standard" contract, he or she is either misrepresenting the situation or is misinformed.

You have developed an incredible amount of knowledge about and experience in your specialty, but that specialty is the practice of medicine – not the business of medicine. You are about to sign the biggest deal of your life. This book's purpose is most definitely not to encourage you to "do it yourself." Instead, I want you to understand the basics, so that when you engage an attorney you are fully aware of the importance of the points the attorney is negotiating on your behalf. Just as your patients will enjoy better outcomes if they become involved in their medical care, you will enjoy a better legal outcome if you are knowledgeable about your contract's key aspects.

 Just as your patients will enjoy better outcomes if they become involved in their medical care, you will enjoy a better legal outcome if you are knowledgeable about your contract's key aspects.

You aren't the right doctor for every patient and every ailment. You have likely concentrated on mastering a relatively small field of medicine and will call in a specialist for issues outside your expertise. By the same token, don't rely on a jack-of-all-trades lawyer in this important negotiation. Be certain to engage an attorney who concentrates his or her practice on physician employment agreements.

Most importantly, don't ever make oral commitments to the recruiter or anybody else you are dealing with. Nobody doubts your ability to be quick and decisive in medical situations. Don't feel that you need to demonstrate these qualities in contract negotiations. Even experienced physicians' attorneys won't make a snap commitment – they will always state any agreement is conditional, based on a review of the documents.

Thus, don't put yourself in the position of feeling that you can't let your attorney negotiate a point that he or she says is unfavorable because you have already conceded that point. Always defer discussions of substantive provisions of your agreement to your counsel, rather than attempting to handle negotiations yourself. The "dumb doc" who claims ignorance of "all that legal stuff" often gets the best overall contract, without straining his or her relationship with future colleagues.

Letters of Intent (Also Known As "Term Sheets")

The contracting process for physician employment agreements frequently (but not always) begins with a letter of intent (sometimes referred to as a "term sheet.")

A letter of intent or term sheet is simply a very brief summary of the main terms of what the parties assume will be a binding formal contract. The purpose of a letter of intent is to make sure that both parties are "on the same page" regarding the major terms of the agreement they hope to form. If you think you're going to be paid $300,000 a year but the employer is expecting to pay $200,000 a year, there may not be any value in continuing negotiations.

You can think of a letter of intent as a means of making sure that it is worthwhile to continue negotiations. Since the purpose of a letter of intent is just to determine if further negotiations are in order, the terms in a letter of intent are generally not legally binding. However, certain provisions of a letter of intent **are** legally binding. Specifically, the letter of intent will most likely provide that each party is responsible for its own attorneys' fees, and that the negotiations will remain confidential. Sometimes a letter of intent will also provide that you will negotiate exclusively with this employer for some period of time. These provisions generally are legally binding (that is, even if you do not sign an employment agreement, you are still bound to pay your own attorneys' fees and keep the terms of the negotiations confidential).

Remember that the purpose of a letter of intent is to make sure that you and your potential employer are on the same page with respect to the major terms of the employment agreement you hope to conclude. Although there will be countless terms and conditions of the final agreement that will be negotiated (you will learn about these later in this book), you should assume that anything you agree to in a letter of intent is "off the table."

Accordingly, your potential employer can be seriously ticked off (sorry for the legal jargon) if you sign a letter of intent that sets forth a specific salary, and then attempt to negotiate a higher salary.

A letter of intent is not a bad way of starting off negotiations for your employment agreement. The employer will generally emphasize that the letter of intent is not legally binding. That is true, but **don't** treat the letter of intent as a meaningless document. If there is something you are uncomfortable with (e.g., the salary offered) you can always attempt to retain flexibility by asking that the hard number be replaced with a phrase such as "an annual salary of approximately $X, to be determined in the definitive physician employment agreement."

Chapter 1: Big Debts, Big Paydays – *(Compensation and Benefits)*

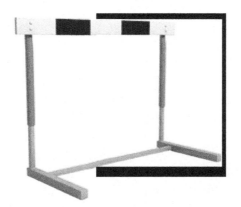

Chapter One

You've worked hard to get where you are. Now it's time to reap the rewards from all that hard work.

Most physicians put tremendous pressure on themselves to succeed. You probably do too. Now, after all those years of training, you may be driven by more than just that usual motivation to succeed. You likely have hundreds of thousands of dollars in student loans. While you were in training, those ever-increasing debts may have seemed almost like Monopoly money (that is, not real), even if all those zeros were a little hard to ignore.

The fact that probably allowed you to sleep at night was that the loans wouldn't be due until you got out of training (a time that, no doubt, seemed to be an eternity away). Now you are about to begin to repay those massive debts.

Given the numbers involved, the first offer you get is likely going to knock your socks off. The new employer will happily pay you many multiples of what you have been earning in training. So, it's all good, right?

Well, maybe, or maybe not. Compensation plans come in a variety of shapes and sizes. Figuring out if the salary offered is appropriate is much more complicated than simply asking your classmates what they have been offered. A physician with the same specialty will receive different compensation in Manhattan than in Boise.

Perhaps more importantly, employers expect to "get what they pay for," so to speak. If two employers in close geographical proximity offer substantially different base salaries (let's assume the other benefits are roughly the same), you can bet your bottom dollar that the employers have different productivity expectations. If you haven't learned it yet, now is a good time to realize that there is no such thing as a free lunch. (Recruitment lunches may be an exception to this rule, depending on how you look at things.)

The employer offering the higher salary is probably expecting you to work harder than the employer offering a lower salary is. That may be perfectly fine with you – some physicians are willing to keep knocking themselves out to get the golden ring. However, many physicians have lifestyle goals that are incompatible with long hours and super-efficient patient contact goals. For these physicians, an employer offering a lower salary might be a better long-term choice.

That's why an analysis of the proposed compensation plan (to give you an accurate idea of how a given compensation package stacks up against benchmarks in the geographical area) is so important. This analysis can calculate how much productivity a compensation package probably implies.

A compensation analysis is included as an integral part of the Physician Prosperity Program®, but one can be obtained separately from many practice consultants too.[1] Just be sure you work with a knowledgeable consultant who has access to the relevant benchmarks. A good consultant will also explain the limitations of various benchmarks, including small sample size and other variables.

PRODUCTIVITY COMPENSATION

Not that many years ago, every new physician received a guaranteed base salary. Frequently, some sort of productivity incentive program accompanied this base. Today, the vast majority of employers still provide a guaranteed salary, but the amount of the guarantee and the length of the guarantee period are eroding as employers feel the pinch of declining reimbursement.

In my opinion, an employer should not bring on a new physician unless that employer is certain that there is sufficient demand to keep that physician busy. I don't believe the risk of acquiring enough work should fall upon the new physician's shoulders. Unfortunately, you will find there are employers willing to take a chance on hiring a new physician and "cover their bets" by shifting the risk of

---

[1] For information about the Physician Prosperity Program®, please visit https://PaHealthLaw.com

insufficient work to physicians through compensation plans based largely (or even completely) on the physicians' productivity.

 Some employers shift the risk of insufficient work to physicians through compensation based on productivity.

At law firms, the method of paying lawyers based upon the business they personally bring in is called "eat what you kill." For obvious reasons, this terminology is rarely used at medical practices. However, the "eat what you treat" compensation method is becoming increasingly common in physician contracts, so you must understand how it can affect you.

At first blush, the concept of paying you based on your productivity hardly seems unfair. After all, if you're not pulling your weight, why should you bring in the big bucks? If there is sufficient work to keep you busy, then it seems completely appropriate to penalize you if you are unable or unwilling to perform at the same level as your colleagues are.

You know that the practice of medicine requires total dedication. You also know that patients cannot be treated if they are not examined. What you don't know is how many patients are going to present themselves to any given practice. The hottest practice in town (including a hospital practice) can get hammered when a "competitor" (yes, this term is used in the medical field, especially by hospitals) hires a superstar physician or buys the latest medical gizmo.

I have seen practices decimated when one physician becomes impaired, especially when a physician has a spectacular burnout. I have been involved in situations in which a surgeon was ejected from the operating room because a nurse smelled alcohol on his breath. In another instance, a security camera picture of a physician breaking into the drug cabinet was introduced into evidence. I can also recall a physician being called to sign a death certificate at a nursing home and doing what apparently was supposed to be a comedy routine, which involved treating the corpse as a puppet – in front of the grieving family.

All of those examples could be expected to raise doubts within the community about the practice that the impaired physician is (or was) associated with. When patients or referral sources become leery of a practice, patient volume can be drastically reduced. Such a reduction will impact the less senior physicians most dramatically. The senior physicians are likely to have a patient base that will still come in no matter what another physician in the practice may have done (or been accused of doing). The less senior physicians, those who are building their reputations and practices, get hit the hardest in these scenarios.

I passionately believe that an employer should base the bulk of a new physician's compensation on a guaranteed salary. Of course, the contract can include protections for the employer if the physician isn't working. For example, most contracts will allow an employer to terminate employment without cause upon reasonable notice, so a turn in fortunes won't doom the employer to paying a salary when you simply aren't working very hard (whether it is your fault or not).

That said, basing your pay on productivity after a few years of employment is not as egregious as agreeing to "eat what you treat" as a new physician. At some point, you can reasonably be expected to develop your own practice. You just shouldn't be required to do so the first day on the job.

Productivity compensation formulas can be extremely complex. However, complexity isn't necessarily a bad thing, as long as the formula is understandable and internally consistent.

TYPES OF PRODUCTIVITY FORMULAS

Productivity formulas tend to be based on either billings, collections or Relative Value Units (RVUs). Formulas based on billings or collections are generally simpler than RVU-based formulas.

FORMULAS BASED ON BILLINGS OR COLLECTIONS

Formulas based on billings or collections typically pay you some percentage of billings or collections for the work you have performed. For example, a collection-based formula could pay you x% of all collections from your work.

To encourage you to work harder, these formulas often provide a higher percentage of collections after a set dollar amount. I have seen many variations of formulas that provide x% of collections up to the first $x of collections per year, and x+y% of collections over $x. In these cases, the set dollar amount is often what the employer assumes the total cost of the physician will be to the practice. Assuming a given employer has a 50% overhead, a physician with a salary of $150,000 is likely to cost the employer $300,000 in salary, benefits, staff support, rent, and so forth in a year. A hypothetical formula for that employer could pay you 30% of collections up to the first $300,000 in collections per year and 35% of collections in excess of $300,000 per year.

Be aware that basing compensation on collections puts you at the mercy of the employer's billing capabilities. While private practices tend to do an excellent job of collecting for physician services, health systems are notorious for inefficient physician billing. (If you think about it, the time of an accounts receivable clerk at a hospital is probably better spent chasing six-figure ICU bills, rather than two or three-figure physician bills.) Basing compensation on billed services (rather than collections) eases that concern slightly, but it also makes auditing the calculation more difficult. Some small private practices can't (or won't) calculate billed services – their books show full, billed charges until the payor pays. At that time, the charge is adjusted downward to the contractual allowance with that payor for those services.

As we'll discuss in greater depth below, you may additionally be providing administrative services that are valuable to the employer but don't generate any revenue directly.

FORMULAS BASED ON RVUS

RVUs are designed to rank the resources used to provide services to patients. Medicare, for example, uses three separate RVUs to calculate the fees paid to providers However, virtually all physician productivity formulas are based on just one of these RVUs: the physician work RVU (or "wRVU"). Although the payment calculation for RVUs is somewhat controversial, use of these RVUs as a proxy for productivity is common.

One advantage to using wRVUs is that Medicare has promulgated the wRVU value of every patient service that you perform as a physician, and these wRVUs are tied to the CPT billing codes used. Therefore, it is relatively easy for an employer to calculate your wRVUs.

Another advantage to the wRVU system of productivity calculation is that it doesn't penalize you for your patient mix. An initial consultation for a new patient has the same wRVU value for every patient: charity, self-paying, or private insurance patients all generate the same wRVUs for the same service. For this reason, wRVU formulas are most commonly seen in hospital settings, especially at nonprofit hospitals, which have a mission to provide community healthcare regardless of individuals' ability to pay.

The problem with wRVU-based formulas is that they only tally patient encounters. This has especial relevance for physicians in the hospital setting, who are likely to be "asked" to take on numerous administrative roles. Those roles include committee assignments, review of budget and new equipment requirements, and medical director duties. If the hospital is entering a new service line and you are the first physician in that specialty, you could even end up being the department head. The hospital will also expect you to be active on the medical staff.

All of these duties provide value to the employer but do not have any wRVUs associated with them. For that reason, some wRVU-based formulas have rather complex mechanisms to extend physicians credit for administrative duties. Since Medicare hasn't promulgated wRVUs for those duties, it is up to you and your employer to negotiate how such service factors into productivity calculation, or if you should be separately compensated for administrative duties (my preference).

THE BOTTOM LINE

As I said before, I don't think basing a new physician's compensation completely on productivity is reasonable. The employer should decide whether a new doctor can be kept busy before making him or her an offer. That decision should factor in the risk that the new physician may not be completely productive at first. This risk of potential loss should be borne by the employer, not the new physician, who probably will have little or no control over how many patients the employer will have, or how many of those patients will be assigned to each physician.

Any employer that bases your pay on productivity must allow for reasonable review of the numbers on which a productivity calculation is based. I have dealt with many physicians being compensated by a formula who are simply presented with a "report" that indicates what the employer feels they are entitled to. In many instances, they begin keeping their own records of, for example, patients seen, and discover that the employer's figures are understated. However, other than increasing the frustration level, the physician's records are likely to be of little use if the employment agreement does not provide them with the right to audit or adjust the employer's figures.

BONUS COMPENSATION

After my ranting about the evils of productivity compensation, you might think I am opposed to any method of calculating compensation that bases pay on productivity. That's only true, though, to the extent that your base compensation (especially in the first year or two) is based on "eat what you treat."

Many employers will still pay a reasonable base salary and then provide productivity "kickers," or bonuses, on top of that salary if goals are met. Giving such bonuses is a great way for employers to compensate physicians for making efforts beyond what is expected of them. Of course, the bonus formula must be clear and unambiguous, and you need the ability to confirm numbers presented by the employer.

I often run into bonus calculations (especially from hospitals and academic institutions) that provide for an annual "reset" of the bonus formula. There is little you can do to protect yourself in such a situation – you just have to hope that the political processes in the department will work appropriately to protect the interests of all the physicians involved.

In general, you should assume that you will not qualify for any bonus offered. Too many physicians get seduced into positions with "adequate" pay, based on promises of tens (or even hundreds) of thousands of dollars they "should" earn from the bonus offered. Unless you will be working in Lake Wobegon, you can't assume everyone is above average.[2] A compensation analysis on the proposed bonus should reveal how the threshold(s) for earning the bonus compare to benchmarks.

---

[2] With apologies to Garrison Keillor.

Too many physicians accept "adequate" pay because they are lured in by big bonuses. However, unless you're in Lake Wobegon, don't assume everyone is above average.

SIGN-ON BONUSES AND MOVING EXPENSES

There is a definite trend toward paying new physicians sign-on bonuses. If a sign-on bonus isn't included in an employer's initial offer, I always ask for one. Such bonuses can range from $10,000 to over $125,000.

In addition, many larger employers reimburse relocation expenses. Sometimes they even offer a housing allowance to compensate physicians for losses sustained in selling their homes in a down real-estate market – although senior physicians who own homes tend to find this perk more interesting than their younger counterparts.

Some physicians leaving training for their first position can pack all of their belongings into their car, so the relocation bonus is effectively wasted on them. In some cases, though, I have been able to persuade an employer to decrease the relocation expense reimbursement and increase the sign-on bonus. Although there used to be a tax advantage to characterizing money received as a relocation allowance, recent tax law changes have removed this advantage, so a sign-on bonus and a relocation reimbursement have the same tax effect.

It is common for the initial offer to stipulate that the sign-on bonus and/or relocation expense reimbursement must be repaid if employment is terminated before the agreement's initial term ends. Most of those provisions provide for what is called an "amortization" of the repayment obligation. In other words, the agreement may provide that you must repay a fraction of the bonus if you leave before the end of the initial term; the bonus fraction is based on the fraction of the time you didn't work there. For example, if the initial term is for three years (36 months) and you leave after 12 months, the agreement could provide that you would keep 12/36 of the bonus, but must repay the balance (24/36) of the bonus.

Relocation expense bonuses are generally a reimbursement of money you actually paid. For that reason, I try to avoid any repayment obligation for your moving expenses that the employer reimbursed.

You should be protected if the employer terminates your employment without cause, if you terminate the agreement because the employer breached it, or if the agreement is terminated because of your death or disability. In such cases, you should not have to repay the bonus.

Finally, I have been able to negotiate a shorter amortization period for some physicians. Let's return to the above example. Say, in that case, that the employer agrees that you must only repay a portion of the bonus if employment is terminated before the first 12 months of the agreement. If that deal is in place, you would not have to repay any part of your bonus if you stick around for a year or more.

Sometimes the sign-on bonus and/or the relocation expense reimbursement are structured as a loan, where you sign a promissory note and agree to repay the amounts advanced if you don't stay a given period of time. If that is the case, you should realize that you may recognize taxable income in the years the "loan" is forgiven. Let's say you receive a $30,000 sign-on bonus that is structured as a loan on December 31, 2020. If the agreement provides that the loan will be forgiven over two years, you would have the following taxable income reported: 2020 - $0; 2021 – $15,000; 2022 - $15,000.

This is not a bad deal for you (if the bonus had not been treated as a loan, you would have paid the full tax on the bonus in 2020). You just have to be aware that your taxes will be going up in the next two years, even though you won't have received any cash. Avoid a nasty tax surprise in the years the loan is forgiven by increasing your tax withholding to account for this "phantom income."

OTHER BENEFITS

Although not as immediately appealing as cash compensation, other benefits (disability pay, health insurance, and retirement benefits, etc.) are major pieces of your compensation package and each should be carefully analyzed. Unfortunately, only a few aspects of the benefits package generally will be open for negotiation.

DISABILITY PAY

Disability pay is one area in which I have been able to obtain concessions from employers. Two aspects of disability pay warrant your attention.

First, analyze the employer's definition of disability and method of determining it. A physician who is mutually agreeable both to the employer and to you should determine disability. You will be working for one or more physicians, and you don't want to find yourself in a situation wherein your boss can unilaterally declare you to be disabled (and therefore unable to work). Sometimes an employer will sidestep this issue by stipulating that an employee is considered disabled for employment agreement purposes when that employee's disability insurance treats him or her as disabled. This alternative is better than allowing the employer to determine disability, but it is not as good as stipulating that a mutually agreeable physician will make the determination.

Second, look at how long (if at all) your employer will pay you if you become disabled. Some employers can be persuaded to provide full pay for some period (usually no more than three or four months), then providing a fraction of your pay for an extended time. For example, I have negotiated packages in which a disabled physician would receive three months of full pay, then three months of half pay, and then three months of one-quarter pay. I have also negotiated longer periods of full pay, such as six months, followed by no pay.

31

HEALTH INSURANCE

The employer almost certainly has a health insurance plan and will be unable to change the details of the coverage provided in the contract. For example, if the plan has a $20 deductible, the employer will be unable to change that provision for you, no matter how badly its physicians want you. Regarding health insurance, the important points to look at are the following: first, whether your dependents will be covered at no additional cost to you; and second, the overall cost-sharing that the employer will expect from you.

A small employer may be willing to include dependent or family coverage as part of the deal, but the attitude to most other elements of health insurance benefits tends to be, "Take it or leave it." That isn't a tough negotiation tactic – the employer and its employees all are subject to the terms of the policy purchased.

Larger employers' "insurance" may be "self-funded" (that is, the employer pays for the costs of medical care out of its general funds). However, even if the employer is providing the "insurance", coverage will be subject to a formal written plan that the employer will probably not be able to alter.

To examine cost sharing, you should request a copy of the plan's Summary Plan Description (SPD). If you are looking at two potential employers, a comparison of their plans' SPDs will give you a good idea of the benefits' differences.

DISABILITY INSURANCE

Here again, the SPD will be the best guide to the benefits an employer has offered you. Since most employers purchase insurance for long-term disability, these provisions are unlikely to have any "give."

Nevertheless, you should confirm that the disability policy defines a disability as an inability to work in your own occupation. That simply means that you are considered disabled (and therefore eligible for benefits) if you are unable to practice medicine. (Some policies go even further, allowing for partial disability based on inability to perform procedures.)

Beware of policies that define disability as the inability to hold gainful employment. As a college graduate, you very well might be able to manage a McDonald's restaurant even if you can't practice medicine. If you don't believe that getting free fries for the rest of your life makes all that education worthwhile, avoid relying on a policy like that.

Again, you most likely won't be able to change the nature of the disability insurance policy an employer has offered. Instead, the purpose of analyzing disability policies is to compare packages offered by competing employers and to see if you might need to purchase a separate policy that will provide the protection you need.

VACATION, CME, ETC.

Although some specialties get more vacation time than others, you should not accept less than two weeks of paid vacation and one week of paid time off for continuing medical education in the agreement's initial year. Some specialties have considerably more vacation, and two weeks of CME is not unheard of – especially if you practice in a sub-specialty or are double-boarded. National benchmarks are useful to determine what is standard for your specialty. For more senior physicians, the amount of paid time off should increase. The employer should also pay all or some portion of the CME costs. I have been able to negotiate additional paid time off for board certification/recertification testing, as well as payment by the employer for the costs associated with board certification and recertification.

If you are required to maintain hospital privileges, the employer should agree to pay for your medical staff dues. In addition, some employers are willing to pay for Drug Enforcement Administration (and/or state equivalent) fees, cell phones and usage plans, and mileage allowances for trips between offices or to the hospital or other facilities.

Many employers will pay your dues to the American Medical Association or the American Osteopathic Association, and/or to state and local medical societies. Frequently, employers also pay dues on your behalf to one or more specialty societies.

It is also becoming more common for employers to agree to pay a portion of your medical school debt. That repayment can take different forms: for example, some employers might offer a flat monthly payment or an annual payment at the end of each contract year. These repayments can total $75,000 or more.

Although less common, some employers will agree to pay you a monthly residency or fellowship stipend between the time you execute the agreement and the time you start work.

It's always worth asking for a private office – although it seems these are becoming less common all the time for new physicians. If you are in a surgical specialty, you can sometimes obtain guarantees about reasonable blocks of time in the OR. Finally, it is sometimes possible to negotiate the right to have input into hiring or firing of support staff (such as nurses, LPNs, and others).

Every benefit package will be different. Don't expect all the benefits listed above from any one employer. At the same time, it never hurts to ask about these benefits. The meek may inherit the earth, but they rarely obtain the best compensation packages.

 It never hurts to ask about specific benefits. The meek may inherit the earth, but they rarely obtain the best compensation packages.

THE CLAUSE THAT WILL MAKE YOU NUTS

As if it isn't bad enough that an employer won't (and probably can't) negotiate various benefit plans' terms, employment agreements almost universally contain a clause that gives the employer the unilateral right to change the benefit plans at any time. That's just a reflection of reality. If the insurer changes a policy's terms, the employer will either be stuck with those changes or will want to change insurers or policies. The employer has to retain discretion in its contract with you in order to change your benefits without your consent.

Although the employer may be stuck with whatever the insurance companies throw at it regarding some benefit plans, you want to make sure that the employer's discretion to change your benefits only applies to the benefit plans that the employer is purchasing from a third party or is offering as part of a tax-qualified plan (such as retirement benefits).

Many agreements list all employee benefits on a separate schedule from the agreement, and then the agreement provides that the employer may amend that schedule unilaterally at any time. Such a provision is acceptable for health insurance, disability insurance, and qualified plans, etc. However, the schedule should not include vacation, CME allowances, sign-on bonuses, or anything else that the employer is not relying on a third party to provide.

WHO IS PAYING FOR THESE BENEFITS?

Sometimes an employment agreement will set forth a decent list of benefits; however, it will then provide that those benefits are part of the physician's overhead and are charged directly against that physician in the compensation calculation. This is unusual, though, outside of agreements based on productivity (or owners' employment agreements in private practices).

Formulas like this are great for private practice owners, since the formulas provide a way to pay personal expenses as part of the practice's tax deductions without becoming taxable to physicians. For example, imagine three partners pay themselves an equal modest salary, but base most of their compensation on a productivity formula that charges expenses against them. If one of the partners wants to take CME courses in Hawaii, the practice can deduct expenses for the CME (along with travel, accommodations, and so forth), while the partner doesn't pay any tax on the payments. At the same time, the spending doesn't harm the other partners, since the costs are charged against the partner who is incurring the expenses and reduce that partner's compensation.

This formula isn't so great for a new physician, though, since that individual's earnings might be erratic in the first year or so. The cost of malpractice insurance for some specialists, in particular, can make up a huge percentage of a first-year physician's salary. Basing gross compensation on productivity for the first year of employment is bad enough, but charging the employer's overhead costs to a new physician is even worse. This is another reason I don't like to base a first-year physician's compensation solely on a productivity formula.

MONEY YOU DON'T WANT

Fraud and abuse laws (predominately the federal Anti-Kickback Statute and the Stark Law, although many states have adopted versions of these laws) generally prohibit paying or receiving payment for referrals of recipients of government-funded health benefits. Penalties for these "tainted" claims range from fines and recouping of money paid to jail time. Regulations interpreting these laws, which constitute thousands of pages, attempt to outline every possible way a devious provider could circumvent these prohibitions.

I would not expect you to encounter an employer who deliberately intends to violate those laws. Yet, because the laws are so complex, I have seen many agreements that a regulator could construe as violating the law. You might expect this issue would be confined to small, private practices that are trying to save legal fees. However, I have also reviewed hospital system agreements that had not been updated to reflect the latest regulations and therefore could expose both the hospital and the physician to liability.

These laws are subtle and complicated; they require expert legal counsel. For example, I once reviewed a private practice's employment agreement that required a new

38

physician to cover all the practice's hospitalized patients, regardless of which practice physician had admitted the patient. The practice made a good-faith effort to compensate the new physician for these extra duties by offering to pay him all the profits from any pathological lab work (performed by the practice) he ordered for these patients while they were inpatient. I assume that the profits from the lab work would constitute reasonable compensation for the time and hassle of driving to the hospital and seeing these patients.

The problem with this good-faith payment is that it would unquestionably violate fraud and abuse laws. A regulator would describe this type of compensation as payment for referrals of lab work to the practice, which would be a violation for both the practice and the physician. In this case, we politely declined this form of compensation and pointed out concerns with fraud and abuse laws. Ultimately, I worked out a system that compensated for these extra duties without subjecting the physician to the risk of prison time. If we had not been able to make this arrangement, our only recourse would have been to simply forgo the extra compensation – or walk away from the position altogether.

People often ask me if the employer can actually enforce a particularly onerous provision in an employment agreement. An unlawful provision such as the one just described could not be enforced in court. However, some provisions in employment agreements, which can drastically affect your future, are routinely enforced in court (and even more routinely enforced by market forces). Next, we'll take a look at one of the most far-reaching of those provisions.

Chapter 2: They Can't Enforce That, Can They? *(Restrictive Covenants)*

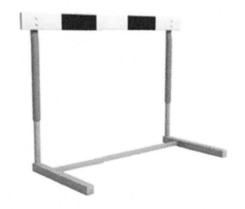

Chapter Two

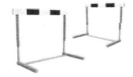

The following has happened more times than I can count. I get a call from a physician, who "has a question about an employment agreement."

I speak to the doctor, who seems a little worried. She is no longer happy with her employer and has been speaking to another employer in the same town. She has a great offer and is ready to give notice.

However, when she pulled out her current contract to see how much notice was required, she detected, as she calls it, a "little problem." The agreement "seems to say" that she can't practice medicine within fifteen miles of her employer's location. Her potential new employer – as well as all three of the local hospitals – is within fifteen miles of her current employer. The upshot of this provision is that she won't be able to practice medicine in this location if she leaves this employer. She will have to move her family and start over. Her children are in school, and she has developed a nice practice here, so leaving town would be traumatic for both her family and her career.

Her question is simple: "They can't enforce that, can they?"

I pause, take a deep breath, and break the news to her as diplomatically and gently as possible: "Unfortunately, they probably can."

Provisions in an employment agreement imposing restrictions on what you can do when you leave employment are called "restrictive covenants." As many physicians, including the doctor described above, have learned the hard way, these provisions can have an enormous impact on your career's course.

Many physicians assume that their first position will end up being where they practice until retirement. In fact, changing employers at some point in a physician's career is becoming more common all the time. Sometimes the charming Dr. Jekyll who interviewed you turns out to be a real Mr. Hyde in day-to-day dealings. Sometimes hospital administration changes and a ruthless cost-cutter who views the medical staff as adversaries replaces the physician-friendly chief executive officer. Finally, sometimes your personal circumstances change and you no longer want to put in the kind of hours expected by your employer.

There are many reasons you may want to change employers at some point in your career. Before you sign anything, make sure you'll be able to make a living at the same location if things don't work out with this employer.

 Before you sign anything, make sure you'll be able to make a living at this particular location if things don't work out with this employer.

WHY DOES SOCIETY ALLOW SUCH RESTRICTIONS?

Many physicians (especially new ones) feel that doctors should never be restricted in where they can practice. They speak of the physician shortage in this country and the difficulty that many patients encounter in just finding a physician. Why in the world would society allow restrictions on medical services when we don't have enough doctors to go around?

To get a better handle on why restrictive covenants are allowed in physician employment agreements, you have to put yourself in the employer's shoes. When you come out of training and see your first patient, whom do you think that patient is coming to see?

Most new physicians' first patients (especially during the first year) probably came to see, or were referred to see, a more senior physician. Faced with the choice of waiting to see their preferred physician in a few weeks or a new physician (you) almost immediately, they chose you. In time you will grow your practice, and patients will want to see you (or referring physicians will refer patients to you). However, when you are starting out, you generally are seeing somebody else's patients.

Having spent time and money to introduce you to the community and local referring physicians, your employer doesn't want you to walk out the door and take those patients or referral sources with you. If you think about it, that position really isn't an unreasonable one.

Even so, you still have to protect yourself against being forced by your contract to move out of town and to start over if things don't work out with your employer. Before agreeing to any restrictive covenant, make sure it is reasonable.

Restrictive covenants have two main components: the geographical area(s) in which you are restricted and the restriction's time period. As you will see, geographical area is generally the more important consideration.

HOW LONG DOES THE PROHIBITION LAST?

A restrictive covenant's two components essentially boil down to time and place. For most physicians, time restrictions are not as important as place restrictions. If you are unable to treat patients for a year (which is the minimum time period agreed upon by most employers), most of your patients will be forced to see another physician. I've found that there isn't much of a difference to you between a one-year and five-year restriction. In either case, you will probably be forced to develop a patient base all over again: in effect, you'll have to start your career over.

When I negotiate these agreements, I try to limit the restricted time to either the time you worked for that employer or one year, whichever is less. However, I often recommend extending the time period if I can obtain a reasonable geographical area and sensible language concerning the restrictions.

WHAT AREA DOES THE PROHIBITION COVER?

Many physicians feel that a restriction's geographical area is more important than the time the restriction lasts. When I'm negotiating agreements, I try to limit the restricted area to no more than a five-mile radius around the employer's office location. In rural areas, a somewhat larger area may be reasonable. (If your patients routinely drive ten miles to the grocery store, a medical office five miles from the old office may be the practical equivalent of an office across the street to an urban employer.) A radius greater than five miles may be reasonable for sub-specialists as well, even in an urban area; however, in no event should you be forced to move out of town and start over if a position doesn't work out.

The prohibited area should be based on the office or any other location where you spent most of your time while working for the employer. Some employers attempt to prohibit you from working within a given radius of each location where any of the employer's physicians see patients.

Similarly, the prohibited area should apply only to your new office location, not every location where your new employer has offices (and certainly not every location where your new employer's physicians see patients!).

WHAT ARE YOU PROHIBITED FROM DOING?

The language concerning these restrictions is crucial and therefore requires meticulous examination. The place restriction should be based on your new office's location, not the general "practice of medicine" in the restricted area.

The language on restrictions must be meticulously examined. A restriction should be based on your new office's location, not the general "practice of medicine" in the restricted area.

If major hospitals are within the prohibited area, then prohibitions on the "practice of medicine" or other sweeping prohibitions could force you to move out of town and start over. It is one thing to agree that patients will have to travel five miles from your old office if they want to see you. It is quite another to agree that you won't see patients in nursing homes, hospitals, and ambulatory surgical centers, etc., within the prohibited area, no matter where your office's new location may be.

48

For the same reason, a restrictive covenant generally should not require you to surrender facility privileges if you leave employment. In some circumstances, however, surrender of privileges may be appropriate. For example, if you work for a private practice that owns an ambulatory surgical center (ASC) with a closed staff (i.e., only members of the practice have privileges at the ASC), then it is reasonable to agree to surrender privileges at the ASC if you leave the practice.

Similarly, some hospitals enter into exclusive contracts with a practice in which only that practice provides services in a given department. For instance, radiology and emergency room services are commonly provided by private practices that have exclusive contracts with the hospital. If your former employer had an exclusive contract with the hospital, your privileges at that hospital would end if your employment ended.

You will probably be prohibited from soliciting your patients to see you at a new employer. It is completely understandable for an employer to expect you to refrain from soliciting old patients while you are still treating them at your old place of work, as well as to refrain from calling patients and urging them to transfer their care to your new employer. It is also reasonable for an employer to prohibit you from writing letters that urge patients to follow you.

However, the language of these particular prohibitions can be troublesome. For example, would you be in violation of a provision prohibiting "direct or indirect solicitation of patients" if you or your new employer has a yellow page ad or uses other general media advertisements such as a website? Language such as this should always provide that general media advertisements do not constitute indirect solicitation of patients.

You will also likely be prohibited from "direct or indirect solicitation" of your old employer's employees. Here, again, it is reasonable on the previous employer's part to prohibit you from trying to get that awesome nurse, whom your employer has trained so well, to join you at your new position. However, any such prohibition should clearly exclude general media advertisements, such as "help wanted" ads.

WHEN THE RESTRICTIVE COVENANT SHOULDN'T APPLY

A restrictive covenant should contain provisions that allow you to leave employment under some circumstances without the restrictions that would normally apply. In particular, a restrictive covenant shouldn't apply if an employer terminates you without cause. It's one thing for an employer to uproot you and move you to a new location, only to decide that there just isn't enough patient volume (or that it's not a good fit). It's quite another thing to prevent you from working for anybody else in your new location.

Similarly, a restrictive covenant should not apply if the practice breaches its agreement with you, although it can be difficult to negotiate a provision to that effect. Employers may be concerned that a physician will claim some far-fetched theory of an alleged breach in order to get out of a restrictive covenant. In this situation, an employer's legitimate concern may be alleviated if the parties negotiate a specific list of grounds for the covenant's release. For example, most employers will agree that if you leave because they aren't paying you they shouldn't enforce a restrictive covenant. In addition, many hospitals are willing to waive a restrictive covenant as long as you don't go to work for a competing health system.

Finally, a restrictive covenant should not apply if you go to work for an employer that does not compete with your current employer – for example, a Veterans Administration facility.

MONEY FIXES EVERYTHING (SOMETIMES)

Some employers will let you "buy out" of a restrictive covenant. The price is rarely low. Walking away from the employer and continuing to practice within the prohibited area will probably cost you at least a year's salary.

If the employer is willing to discuss a buyout, the price should preferably decline over time. There are two reasons that a reduction of the buyout over time is reasonable.

First, if you leave in the first year or so of employment, you probably will be taking along lots of patients who really "belong" to the employer (i.e., patients who came to the practice to see a more senior physician but were assigned to you). However, after a few years at a practice, you will probably have your own referral base. Consequently, most of the patients who will go with you most likely came to your old employer initially to see you specifically.

Second, the employer will have recouped its investment in you after some period of time. Bringing in a new physician means that the employer would incur recruiting costs and credentialing costs. The employer likely also will endure a period in which the new doctor's salary is more than the amount he or she generates. This initial slow period may be a result of insufficient demand, delays in obtaining payment from managed care payors, or both.

For these reasons, physicians can sometimes negotiate a reduction in the buyout price of a restrictive covenant.

THE BOTTOM LINE ON RESTRICTIVE COVENANTS

A restrictive covenant is one of the most important aspects of your employment agreement. Never count on a covenant being unenforceable. Always assume that if you leave the employer, the restrictive covenant will apply. If it does apply, you should focus on determining whether you would be able to remain in that location and practice medicine.

I have represented several physicians who signed covenants so outrageous that they likely would be difficult to enforce in court. These physicians learned the hard way that new employers are leery of hiring a physician who comes with a built-in lawsuit – no matter how likely that the lawsuit would eventually be found to be without merit. A former employer attempting to stop a physician's defection could sue that physician for breaching the restrictive covenant and might also sue the physician's new employer for "intentional interference with contractual relations."

One particularly egregious example illustrates this point well. I once represented a physician who signed a non-compete covenant that prohibited the practice of medicine within 65 miles. That physician was courted by a hospital roughly 62 miles from his former employer. We realized early in the contract negotiations that this ludicrous covenant existed. Even though the hospital's legal counsel and I agreed that the old employer would almost certainly not prevail if it sued, the hospital decided not to hire a physician with that sort of baggage. The offer was revoked.

As you can see, it's essential that you get a clear picture of what will happen and what you will and will not be able to do if you decide to leave your employer. Next, we'll talk about an equally vital aspect of an agreement – what you are required to do while you are employed.

Chapter 3: I'll Have to Work When and Do What? *(Requirements of Employment)*

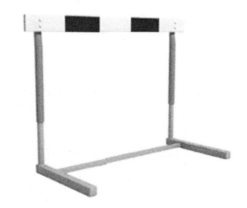

Chapter 3: I'll Have to
Work When and Do
WHAT (Requirements
of Employment)

Chapter Three

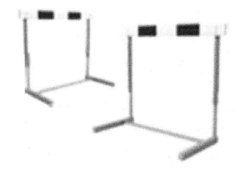

Through are some contract negotiations you never forget. One of my more memorable negotiations involved a new physician, just out of training, who was offered a position at a solo private practice. The practice's current owner was ready to expand and wanted help with his 24/7 call coverage schedule.

Like most first offers, the draft agreement initially presented wasn't perfect – but it didn't seem particularly horrible either. A good contract should be crystal clear on the parties' rights and responsibilities. The offer was a little fuzzy on several points, and I requested that the practice's attorney clear up the ambiguities. One of these fuzzy points was assignment of call coverage.

The draft agreement simply provided that the employer would assign call coverage. There was no mention of how exactly coverage would be assigned. I requested a specific schedule, or, at a minimum, a provision that call coverage would be equitably allocated.

However, when the other side presented their first proposed revision, the offending language was left unchanged. The practice's attorney rather sheepishly explained that his client wasn't willing to agree to allocating call coverage equitably. Since the solo physician had been practicing alone for six years, doing 24/7 coverage, he intended to assign 24/7 coverage to the new physician, "at least for the first few years." The attorney was concerned that there "could be an argument" that this contemplated arrangement wasn't equitable.

Needless to say, more negotiations were in order. We eventually convinced the owner that he would never get anybody to help him unless he was willing to share call coverage. If we hadn't straightened that issue out, my client would have been miserable in her new position.

I can't emphasize this enough: the purpose of a written agreement is to *remove any doubts* about what is expected of you (and what is expected of the employer). Many first offers contain extremely vague language about what is expected of the physician. For example, an initial offer may provide that you are required to work "full time" without defining that term. Larger practices and hospitals may be willing to stipulate specifically that you work 40 hours per week, exclusive of call coverage.

With regard to larger employers, it is important to get a commitment about requirements for patient contact hours. If the employer expects you to have 40 patient contact hours, then you are likely to be working significantly more than 40 hours per week. In particular, if the employer doesn't use hospitalists, you may spend a significant amount of time seeing inpatients.

Some employers initially offer a "40-hour week," which turns out to mean 40 hours of seeing patients in the office. When patients are admitted, rounding is expected to occur outside of those 40 hours. This can be especially onerous if the employer admits patients to multiple hospitals. Of course, you will still be spending considerable time on charting.

Smaller employers are likely to require much more flexibility in scheduling. If a practice or hospital department only has three physicians, for example, call coverage and patient contact hours are likely to spike several times throughout the year. Each time a third of the physicians (i.e., each physician) take vacation or CME time off, the call coverage and patient contact hours will probably significantly increase for the remaining two physicians, who are temporarily doing the work of three.

Call coverage requirements in private practices can also be complicated. Frequently, senior partners will enter a "glide path" into retirement. That is, at some point the senior partner may stop taking call. In a larger private practice, increased call coverage may be negligible for the remaining physicians. However, in a smaller practice, removing one physician from call coverage can have a substantial impact. In these cases, you have to balance the desire for a workable call coverage schedule for the new physician with quality-of-life concerns for the senior physicians. Sometimes the new physician simply has to "pay dues" with the understanding that when that physician is nearing retirement there will be payback.

Larger employers may provide an expected call coverage schedule (e.g., one night every seven and one weekend per month). These schedules will rarely be firm commitments. However, sometimes the employer will agree to stipulate that call coverage will not exceed some limit (e.g., one night in four or two weekends per month).

National benchmarks indicate how much unpaid call physicians in your specialty handle per week. They also provide guidelines for payment when call exceeds those thresholds. When negotiating these agreements, I always try to get the median call compensation for call coverage beyond the median unpaid call per week.

A true 40-hour work week may be attainable if the employer is willing to agree to about 32 patient contact hours each week, inclusive of time spent rounding at hospitals, nursing homes, ASCs, etc. That should give you adequate time to handle charting, medical staff meetings, and other administrative duties – and still have a life outside the practice of medicine.

No matter how well I negotiate provisions concerning call coverage assignments, I have found that the newest physician always seems to end up with call coverage on Christmas. Isn't that a freakish coincidence?

WHEN DO YOU START, AND WHEN DO YOU STOP?

THE BEGINNING

You may feel that your first position is the universe's reward for all your hard work in medical school and beyond, but your employer has a slightly different concept in mind. To be blunt, your employer hired you so that you can generate revenue for them.[3]

That said, many employment agreements provide a starting date but contain conditions that may move that date back. No employer will let you start seeing patients if you haven't obtained a license to practice medicine in that state, for example. Similarly, most employment agreements will require you to have federal DEA (and equivalent state) authority to prescribe medicine. These requirements should not be a problem for most physicians, given the normal timeframe for recruitment and negotiation. As long as you are reasonably diligent in applying, the DEA and most state

---

[3] Of course, nonprofit hospitals are only hiring you to improve healthcare in the community. The phrase "no money, no mission" is never uttered in the sacred halls of their executive suites.

boards of medicine will process your application(s) fairly quickly. Expecting you to be diligent is hardly unreasonable from the employer's perspective.

However, many agreements also impose starting conditions that are at least partially out of your control. One of the most common is the requirement that you obtain hospital privileges and become accepted as a participating provider on major payors' panels. Depending on the timeframe of the agreement's execution and its effective date, this may be a real issue.

If you are executing the agreement in November with an assumed start date of the following July or August, this provision should not pose a problem. However, many agreements are not made final until April or May, with an assumed start date of July or August. Hospital credentialing moves at a snail's pace. Most hospitals require "primary verification" of your training, which means they need an official copy of your transcript directly from the schools and residency programs you attended. They may also require a letter from the director of your residency/fellowship program(s). Obtaining those documents can take months.

Once the documents are obtained, one or more committees will examine the files; then, they may want more information (elaboration on a less-than-ringing endorsement from the residency program director, for example). Although the hospital will have paid staff handling the credentialing file's organization, physicians who are already on staff in the relevant department will perform much of the credential analysis – and they are frequently not paid for this thankless task. The hospital staff will generally try to avoid imposing on the physicians any more than necessary, so they won't give committee members a credentials packet until they feel it is complete. The staff will also schedule meetings to be convenient for committee members.

Although it may be a foreign concept to you now, practicing physicians engage in a practice called "vacation," where they frequently hit little balls with expensive sticks at exotic locations. While engaged in this pursuit, these physicians are not available for meetings to look at your credentials. What's worse from your perspective is that there is no "Dean of Vacations" to assure that the physicians all take their vacations at the same time, thereby assuring convenient availability for meetings. Hospital staff members, who are used to working at a snail's pace normally, refer to the summer as a "slow period." If your credentials packet lands at the hospital during the summer, it can take months to get it in front of the committee.

 Normally, hospital staffs work at a snail's pace. If your credentials packet lands at the hospital during the summer "slow period," it can take months to get it to the committee.

As a result of such delays, some physicians with contractual start dates in July, August, or even September find that they have not been granted privileges when they are supposed to start work. They may have moved to town and signed a long-term lease by then, all in anticipation of being employed on the start date. A similar phenomenon can occur with managed care credentials.

The contract provisions regarding what happens if you don't meet the requirements for hospital and managed care credentials become critical if you find yourself in such a situation. You have to recognize the employer's legitimate interest in not being forced to pay you when you aren't able to generate revenue. Nevertheless, you should not be forced to continue in unpaid limbo while the process grinds forward. Negotiations around this issue can be tricky because of the economic importance of the matter to both parties.

First, let's talk about what an agreement should *not* provide. An agreement should not automatically terminate if you aren't credentialed by the effective date, nor should it give the employer the unilateral right to terminate the agreement. Ideally, an agreement should also not simply be suspended until all credentialing is completed.

An agreement should distinguish between a failure to become credentialed and a denial of credentials. If you have been denied hospital credentials, you probably have some major problems in your file; it may be reasonable for the employer to refuse to wait for you to fix those issues. An agreement should also distinguish between failing to obtain credentials because of a lack of responsiveness on your part and failing to obtain credentials because the hospital or managed care company is slow to process an application. The employer should agree to provide administrative assistance to you in credentialing and to use their "best efforts" to expedite the process. Finally, an agreement should only require credentialing with major payors, not every payor that the employer has had dealings with.

When initially negotiating, I always try to insert a provision requiring both parties to sit down in good faith and attempt to negotiate a mutually satisfactory arrangement allowing the physician to start at the original start date, even if credentialing is not complete. For example, if you have hospital credentials and have been accepted by every major payor of the employer except one, the employer may be able to schedule patients for you who are not covered by the slow payor. This may not be possible if a dominant payor hasn't credentialed you, of course. A failure to be credentialed by Medicare is going to have a lot more impact on a geriatrician than a pediatrician, for example.

If all the payors have credentialed you but the hospital has not, perhaps another physician can admit patients and do rounds until you get privileges. Both parties likely can find creative ways to work out something acceptable if the agreement is flexible enough.

You have to be flexible too. If the employer is willing to make concessions to allow you to start, you must be prepared to make concessions as well – and those might include reduced hours and compensation until all the requirements are met.

THE END OF THE LINE

Nothing lasts forever. In today's chaotic healthcare environment, physicians are increasingly playing musical chairs with their careers. Employers have a legitimate desire to ensure that they can terminate your contract if you turn out to be a lousy physician, or if patient demand just doesn't justify paying you any longer. You need to preserve your options too: you may find you want to leave an employer in order to better your career, improve your quality of life, or both.

Your employment agreement should provide reasonable protection to both you and the employer if either of you fails to live up to the terms of the agreement. The agreement should also provide reasonable flexibility for both parties to get out of the deal, even if the other party didn't do anything wrong.

In legal jargon, the phrase "with cause" (or "for cause") refers to termination of the employment agreement because the other party breached it. A party can terminate the agreement for cause if the other party didn't do what it was supposed to do or, alternatively, did something it wasn't supposed to do. A party can also terminate the agreement "without cause" (or "not for cause") even though the other side didn't do anything wrong.

FOR CAUSE TERMINATION

The first draft agreement typically contains numerous grounds that authorize for cause termination for the employer, but not for you, the employee. The reasons you can terminate the agreement because the employer was at fault are usually somewhat limited. In general, simply preserving your right to terminate the agreement if the employer breaches it (i.e., without listing the various ways that might happen) will be enough protection. This will allow you to terminate the agreement if, for example, the employer fails to pay you or fails to do something else that it agreed to do. A skilled physician's contract attorney may obtain the right for you to terminate for cause if the employer is excluded from any federal healthcare program (e.g., Medicare, Medicaid). This is an important protection, since you can be excluded from these programs if you have a contractual relationship with a party that has been excluded.

The employer, on the other hand, will likely have a veritable laundry list of grounds to terminate your employment for cause. Some are hard to argue with, such as if you die or are convicted of a felony. Your ability to see patients will be severely limited if you are in the Great Beyond or behind bars. Similarly, if you lose your medical license, you will have little value to the employer.

Like everything else in the agreement, the exact language regarding termination for cause is critical. In this country, one is generally presumed innocent until proven guilty. However, many employers initially stipulate that you may be terminated for cause if you are indicted (i.e., formally charged with a crime). This point can be difficult to negotiate, since the employer's reputation could be severely damaged if the media reports one of its physicians being charged with a serious crime. Nevertheless, it may be worth fighting for the requirement of an actual conviction as grounds for termination. At a minimum, this ground for termination should only apply to felonies or crimes involving alleged healthcare fraud – you shouldn't lose your job because of a speeding ticket.

A similar argument can be made for loss of hospital privileges. If you actually lose your privileges, then obviously your value to the employer is significantly diminished (and there are probably questions regarding your competence in treating patients, as well). However, initiation of the process to revoke your privileges should not trigger termination of your employment. Medical staff politics can be ugly, and some physicians are not above questioning competence for competitive reasons.

There should not be any question as to how the provisions regarding grounds for termination apply. Presumably, the fact of your death is not something you and your employer will argue about. An actual conviction and a revocation of staff privileges are also both clear-cut grounds for termination.

However, there are likely to be other grounds for termination that will not be so obvious. Disability, for example, is another common ground for termination. As was

68

discussed in Chapter 1, the definition of "disability" is crucial. The provisions regarding termination because of a disability should be consistent with the provisions regarding compensation during your disability. One thing that you have going for you is the Americans with Disabilities Act. The ADA generally requires the employer to make "reasonable accommodation" to allow you to continue to work even though you are disabled.

It's likely the employer will try to provide other grounds for termination that could be subject to dispute. One fairly common ground for termination is the employer's belief that allowing you to continue to treat patients would endanger those patients' health (think of this as a "crappy doctor" termination). While few would argue that a crappy doc should be allowed to continue to treat patients, the quality of care a physician provides may be hard to measure. Occasionally, I have succeeded in arguing that other provisions in an agreement protect the employer (for example, in a hospital setting, the ability to terminate the physician if privileges are revoked protects the employer). More often, I have had to settle for language that requires the "crappy doc" determination be reasonable and in good faith. Such language gives you some ability to challenge the determination, if necessary.

Employers also frequently insert provisions allowing for cause termination if the reputation of the physician or the employer is adversely affected by something the physician did. It's hard to argue with the theoretical appropriateness of that provision. Yet here, again, it is crucial to insert language assuring that any such determination be reasonable and in good faith. In addition, I am usually able to get the employer's counsel to agree that the reputation of the physician and/or the employer must be "materially" adversely affected by something the physician has done. Picking your nose in front of a patient certainly doesn't enhance your reputation or that of your employer – but it shouldn't be grounds for termination.

It is fairly common to allow the employer to terminate the agreement if you are excluded from a managed care company's panel of providers. Obviously, your exclusion from a major payor's panel would have a huge impact on the employer's finances. However, it is important to limit the employer's right to terminate your employment to instances in which you are excluded from panels of payors that are material to the practice. It is one thing for you to be excluded from participation in the Blues (particularly in an area where they dominate the market). It is quite another to be excluded from Mutual of Podunk[4], when the employer only sees about one patient a year with that insurance. In addition, as insurance companies begin to offer more products with "narrow networks", it is important to ensure

---

[4] I am fairly certain that there isn't an insurance company called Mutual of Podunk. If there is, I humbly apologize for any offense taken. I am sure it is a wonderful company, where caring people do their best to change the world for the better.

that you won't be terminated for reasons other than suspicions regarding the quality of care you provide.

Some for cause termination provisions allow a "cure" period. That is, the provision will allow the breaching party to fix ("cure") the problem within a reasonable time. The time allowed to cure a breach varies from as little as five days to sixty days or more. If the employer is given a cure period, you should generally be given one as well. However, don't expect to be given a cure period for everything. Losses of medical licensure, exclusions from payor panels, and losses of hospital privileges can frequently be appealed, both internally and (sometimes) in the courts. If you are convicted of a felony, you may very well have appeal rights all the way up to the Supreme Court. That doesn't mean that the employer should be required to participate in a work-release program if you get out of the slammer every Wednesday while you are appealing a conviction.

For this reason, most for cause termination provisions provide for immediate termination if the provision is triggered. A for cause termination can have a major impact on your chances to obtain a good position elsewhere. If the termination is based on alleged clinical deficiencies, the employer will be required to report the termination to the National Practitioner Data Bank (NPDB). An NPDB report will not only make it harder for you to obtain employment - it will also impact your ability to obtain hospital privileges and to participate in payor panels.

Because of the devastating impact a for cause termination can have on a physician's career, the provisions of the employment agreement relating to for cause termination must be examined and negotiated.

NOT FOR CAUSE TERMINATION

Ideally, the practice of medicine will be a collegial pursuit. Few would argue that your employer should be able to terminate you if you aren't a good fit with the rest of the physicians. By the same token, you obviously want some flexibility to leave an employer if you get a better opportunity or simply aren't happy with the position. For that reason, your employment agreement should have a without cause termination provision unless you are in the United States on a J-1 visa[5]. Such a provision allows you or the employer to terminate employment even though the other party has done nothing wrong.

As you can see, without cause termination provisions are double-edged swords. They give you the right to leave for no reason, but they also give the employer the right to give you the boot for no reason. Generally, only two major aspects of without cause termination require your attention.

First, the notice period (that is, the time between when the other party is notified of the termination without

---

[5] If you are here on a J-1 visa, as you probably know, termination of the employment agreement will probably require you to leave the country.

cause and the date that the termination becomes effective) should give you adequate time to seek suitable replacement employment. Although 90 days' notice is common, I usually try to obtain 120 days' notice. That gives you a much better chance of locking in a new position without a significant break in your income if the employer terminates your employment. Second, you and the employer should both be given the same notice period. I sometimes see provisions in which the employer can terminate without cause by giving 30 days' notice, but the physician has to give 180 days' notice to terminate without cause. When you see one-sided provisions like that, you have to question whether you really want to work for that employer.

If the employer gives notice of a without cause termination, they frequently retain the right to have you stop work immediately. That provision isn't objectionable, so long as they continue to pay you through the termination date.

As an aside, without cause termination provisions are sometimes used to end employment relationships even though one party really does believe that the other side has breached the agreement. I have sent demand letters to employers setting forth claims that the employer has committed one or more breaches. Experience tells me that the employer is likely to dispute an employee's claims of a breach. In addition, the employer may be given a cure period. So, since my client is usually fed up with the place by then, I frequently also give notice at the same time of a without cause termination. That way, my client and I can be sure we have a certain termination date for the agreement.

It is useful to have a provision that requires your approval of any notice sent to patients in the event of a without cause termination by either party.

OTHER ISSUES

Although the hours of work, call coverage requirements, and termination provisions tend to be the biggest issues in this area, all the terms and conditions of a new job must be examined. Let's take a look at frequent problems I encounter:

MEDICAL RECORDS

Almost every agreement will provide that the employer, rather than you, owns the medical records. That is completely reasonable during the term of your employment. However, many first drafts of agreements also provide that after you leave, the employer will transfer records at your expense to a patient that wants to continue to be seen by you. As a practical matter, most employers do not charge patients for copies of their charts, so the provision is really punitive. I usually attempt to negotiate a provision that patients may request to move their medical records, at the patients' expense.

You should also be given the right of free access to any medical record necessary to defend yourself against any actual or threatened malpractice action or peer-review activity. I also attempt to negotiate a provision that

74

authorizes free copies of any record useful in any legal action – including a legal action between you and the employer. A related issue is the confidentiality you are required to maintain.

Medical records are obviously protected by HIPAA[6] and similar state laws. Although it is reasonable to require you to treat all medical records as confidential, some agreements go so far as to prohibit you from disclosing any information about the employer without prior written permission from the employer. With regard to these provisions, it is important to allow an exception for any information that you are required to disclose pursuant to legal process. I encourage you to sing like the proverbial bird if you are subpoenaed or questioned in any legal process.

ASSIGNMENT OF LOCATION OF SERVICE

Many agreements provide that you will work wherever the employer assigns you to work. That provision is troublesome on many fronts. The obvious concern is that, presumably, you will want to live fairly close to your place of work. If you buy a house in Night Vale and the employer moves you completely to King City (or requires you to see patients in both Night Vale and King City), you could suddenly be faced with a significant commute.[7]

---

[6] The federal Health Insurance Portability and Accountability Act, known by lawyers as the "Healthy Income for Practicing Attorneys Act."

[7] As fans of "Welcome to Night Vale" know, it is theoretically impossible to travel from Night Vale to King City.

This problem is exacerbated if you are paid wholly or partially based on productivity. You aren't generating any revenue while you're commuting. Even if you aren't compensated on productivity, I assume that you would have chosen a career as a long-distance trucker if life on the open road had been your life's ambition.

This provision can be ameliorated if a reasonable limitation is placed upon any distance from a given point (e.g., the hospital or your primary office) that the employer is allowed to assign you to work.

MISCELLANEOUS CONCERNS

I once saw a provision that all e-mail communications from referral physicians must be returned within two hours. Theoretically, if a doctor e-mailed you at 11:30 p.m., your response would be required before 1:30 a.m. Frequently, these "weird" provisions are the result of a prior bad experience on the employer's part. If you can determine the employer's underlying concern, you can often negotiate a more acceptable provision addressing that concern.

Hospital contracting can be especially strange in that regard. Many institutions are willing to agree to provide you with "reasonable staff and equipment" to do your job, "subject to budgetary constraints." Does that mean you will be doing your own scheduling and billing if money gets tight? If you are a radiologist, will you be expected to repair the MRI machine if you want to use it? One hopes the answer to those questions is always, "No!" Accordingly, when negotiating agreements, I try to avoid limitations on the employer's responsibility to provide you with what you need.

I also frequently encounter provisions to the effect that the physician agrees to practice medicine in accordance with the "highest standards." Although I'm sure you are a great doctor, I don't think the employer should attempt to impose any standard on you more stringent than those of the community. The standards in the community are the standards you will be held to in a malpractice action. The concern here is that a plaintiff's attorney could obtain your employment agreement in the discovery phase of litigation and attempt to persuade the jury that your treatment didn't meet the "highest" standards, even though that treatment would be perfectly acceptable in your community.

The employer frequently attempts to retain the right to assign a contract, although the physician is never given that right. Since the employer hired you (and not your cousin Vinny) to do this work, prohibiting you from assigning the agreement is perfectly reasonable. However, I am uncomfortable with giving the employer complete freedom in assigning the agreement. You made a conscious decision to work for this employer in this location. However, it is probably acceptable to allow the employer the right to assign your agreement to one of its affiliates – hospitals are known for constantly reorganizing, and you don't want to be the one standing in the way of a nice bonus for the CEO.

Finally, the employer will want you to agree to adhere to its policies and procedures. This is hardly unreasonable, but you should only be bound by policies and procedures that are provided to you in writing. If possible, I also try to require that the policies and procedures be reasonable. Of course, employers can't agree that things completely out of their control (like hospital and medical staff bylaws) have to be "reasonable" but sometimes they will agree to a standard of reasonableness for things under their control.

The issues discussed in this chapter all can have a major impact on how pleasant (or unpleasant) your position will be. Next, let's look at another aspect of your employment agreement that can have a huge financial impact on your career: malpractice insurance.

Chapter 4: Malpractice Insurance

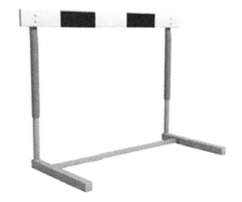

Chapter 4. Malpractice Insurance

Chapter Four

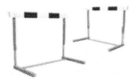

It's a horror story that repeats itself time and time again. A new physician takes a position right out of training and signs the contract presented to her. After a few years, she is ready to move on to greener pastures in another town. She's moving far enough away that her restrictive covenant won't apply, and this time she is getting her offer reviewed by a competent physicians' contract attorney.

Her attorney gives her a thorough written review of the draft contract, and they discuss the review over the phone. One of the lawyer's comments about malpractice insurance puzzles the physician. Her attorney has noted that the new contract contains what he describes as a "common provision," a clause to the effect that the new employer's malpractice insurance will only cover her for claims arising from her new employment. Does her current employer have a "tail"?

The physician is absolutely convinced that her current boss has horns, but she has never seen evidence of a tail. Her attorney explains that a "tail" is a policy that covers the physician for claims that arise after she leaves her current position. Tail coverage isn't always required – depending on the type of insurance her current employer carries, the physician may be covered for those claims automatically. A casual discussion with the office manager at her current position reveals that the practice has claims-made insurance, so the physician will not be covered for any claims that arise after she leaves. Her current contract requires her to purchase tail coverage at her expense when she leaves. The physician is shocked to learn that the premium for tail coverage is about a third of her yearly salary. She reluctantly decides that she can't afford to change jobs now or in the foreseeable future. She is stuck in a position that she hates and has to turn down what seems like a dream job in comparison to her current servitude.

Faced with a staggering insurance cost if she leaves the employer, a doctor turns down a dream job. She feels stuck in servitude.

TYPES OF MALPRACTICE INSURANCE

There are two types of malpractice insurance: occurrence and claims-made policies.

The first type of policy covers you for any claims that "occur" during the period of the policy. If a claim arises based on an alleged action or omission during the period the policy was in force, you are covered – no matter when the action itself arises. In other words, if a case is filed several years after you leave employment, based on alleged malpractice that occurred while you were employed and covered by that policy, you are automatically covered.

The second type of malpractice insurance is claims-made coverage. As the name implies, such a policy will cover only a claim that is made during the policy period (i.e., if a lawsuit is filed or threatened). If you leave employment and a claim is filed against you based on alleged malpractice that occurred while you were employed, this type of policy will not cover you.

There are several reasons an employer may purchase claims-made coverage. First, of course, it is cheaper than occurrence coverage. In addition, sometimes occurrence coverage is simply not an option – occasionally the legal environment reaches a critical mass of craziness, and insurers stop selling occurrence malpractice insurance. As in much of healthcare, these crises tend to be cyclical, so the availability of occurrence insurance varies over time in any given state.

83

To protect yourself after leaving a position where you had claims-made malpractice insurance, you must purchase a separate policy to cover any later claims that are based on alleged malpractice at the old position. This is called "tail coverage."

Tail coverage isn't cheap. Premiums for a "tail" can cost as much as a third of a year's salary. That's why it is so important to make sure your employment agreement addresses payment for a tail when you leave.

Tail coverage isn't cheap – the premiums can cost as much as a third of a year's salary – so make sure your employment agreement addresses which party pays for a tail when you leave.

THE BOTTOM LINE ON MALPRACTICE COVERAGE

The employer should agree to provide malpractice insurance in reasonable amounts. For example, the coverage provided should be no less than the greater of state-mandated minimums or the minimum required for the hospital staffs you are required to join. The type of coverage provided (occurrence or claims-made) is almost never subject to negotiation.

To protect yourself when you leave employment, you have to negotiate responsibility for payment of tail coverage premiums. This must be done regardless of what kind of insurance the employer is currently carrying. Even if the employer has occurrence insurance now, you have to protect yourself if the employer subsequently switches coverage (either voluntarily to reduce costs or because occurrence coverage simply isn't available anymore).

I remember the good old days when virtually every employer was willing to pay for a tail. Those days are long gone. Most hospitals are willing to pay for a tail, although that concession is not uniformly contained in the first offer. Private practices, however, are becoming less likely to offer to pay for tails, especially in the first offer.

I have found that many employers are willing to pay for all or a portion of the tail under certain circumstances, especially if you can convince them that it isn't fair not to pay for a tail. For example, I am frequently able to persuade employers to pay for the tail if they terminate your employment without cause or if employment terminates because of your death or disability.

If I can't get the employer to agree to pay for all of the tail coverage, I am sometimes able to obtain partial payment based on the length of employment. For example, the employer might pay a fifth of the tail's cost for every year of service. That way, if you stick around for five years, the employer pays all the tail's costs.

However, many employers are not willing to pay for any portion of the tail if you terminate employment without cause or if they terminate your employment for cause. Often, I can persuade the employer to pay for some portion of the tail if the agreement provides for partial payment based on length of service (as suggested above), even if the physician *does* terminate the agreement without cause. The employer almost certainly profited from the physician's services over that time, so the employer will often give in on payment for tail if the physician terminates the agreement without cause. However, payment for the tail is a different story when the employer terminates the physician's employment for cause. It's difficult to get the employer to pay for a tail under circumstances in which you really embarrassed the hospital or practice, especially if that embarrassment involved legal exposure.

For those in private practice, the good news is that most practices do pay for a tail for the practice owners. We'll talk about joining that happy club next. (If you are already in the recruitment or negotiation process and are sure you're not going to be working in a private practice, you might want to skip ahead to the Conclusion, where we'll talk about actual negotiations.)

Chapter 5: How Soon Will It Be My Practice? *(Private Practice and Recruitment Agreements)*

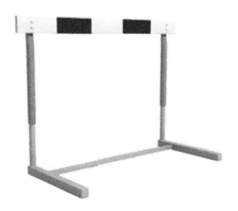

Chapter Five

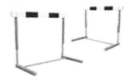

Imagine receiving your first offer from a private practice: it contains a neat little provision concerning your potential ownership. Exciting, right? You can hardly believe your eyes – if you are accepted, it looks as if you will be offered partnership in this apparently very lucrative practice... for just $100! You've seen the partners' houses and cars – there is no doubt that the practice of medicine is treating them very well. The partners seem like nice people, and they obviously like you. You're confident in your abilities; there is no reason to believe you won't be offered partnership. Your biggest concern is that there could be some sort of catch – cue Admiral Ackbar[8].

You obtain a complete review of the agreement from an experienced physicians' contract attorney. Your attorney informs you that, aside from the usual contingencies (e.g.,

---

[8] "It's a trap!" See "Star Wars Episode VI: Return of the Jedi."

there is no guarantee of partnership), the agreement does, indeed, provide for a purchase price of just $100. There is no hidden language, no tricky turn of phrase. Your reading of the clause concerning potential ownership was correct.

You are elated to hear that the attorney's analysis of the buy-in provision matches yours. Then, your attorney tells you that he doesn't like the idea of being able to get a huge chunk of this practice for just $100.

THE TRACK TO THE GOLDEN RING

For most physicians accepting positions at private practices, the time it will take until they become owners is one of the biggest things on their minds. Over my 20+ years of reviewing and negotiating physician employment agreements, I've often been asked what is considered "standard" for a given specialty or location.

I've never been able to answer that question. The time to ownership does not appear to be uniform among specialties, practices of the same general size, or even practices in the same geographical area. I've seen variations in the time until ownership from one to eight years. Other than the general observation that radiologists (and sometimes oncologists) "eat their young" (i.e., practices in these specialties tend to be extremely harsh in treatment of new employees and even junior partners), there does not seem to be a detectable pattern in how long a practice will make you wait before you are offered partnership. Instead, it seems the wait time for most practices is based on the time the founder made the first employed physician wait until he or she was offered partnership.

Concerning those practices that stretch out the time to an offer of partnership, one thing you have going for you is the free-market economy in this country. More experienced physicians have greater opportunities to leave and the ability to command higher salaries elsewhere. This means that the physicians who have to wait longer for an offer of partnership are usually earning almost as much as the owners by the time the offer is presented.

Many physicians feel that the initial employment offer should guarantee partnership. I disagree. The practice of medicine should be collegial. No matter how good you are as a clinician, the owners of the practice need to feel that there is a fit personally. One of the benefits of owning your own practice is the ability to determine who you will (and won't) work with. The factors involved in offering partnership are likely to include much more than someone's clinical abilities.

 A benefit of owning your own practice is choosing who you'll work with – and it's likely that decision will be based on more than someone's clinical abilities.

For this reason, a provision might provide "After x years, you will be considered in good faith" to be offered the opportunity to purchase an ownership interest. That's hardly much assurance to you, as a newly hired physician, but if you want to become a partner you have to start thinking like one. Partners generally want to feel comfortable with their fellow partners.

However, some agreements do guarantee partnership if certain financial goals are met. Those agreements tend to scare me. If your financial performance is the only thing the practice is concerned about, the employer may consider you solely as a commodity. In addition, as I said before, if you want to be a partner, think like one. What if the next physician hired by the practice is a total jerk? Do you really want to spend the rest of your professional career tied to somebody you can't stand just because he or she has strong financial performance?

HOW MUCH IS THIS GOING TO COST ME?

As I've indicated before, it probably isn't in your own best interest to sign a contract that guarantees you partnership. However, even if you aren't guaranteed an opportunity to buy into a practice, the method of determining purchase price if you're offered that opportunity should still be included in your employment agreement.

Even if you aren't guaranteed partnership, the employment agreement should still provide how the purchase price would be determined if partnership is eventually offered.

There are no hard and fast rules regarding how a given practice will value its shares. Each practice seems to put a slightly different spin on the valuation. Still, the methods can generally be divided into three categories: fixed dollar amount, fair market value, and book value.

FIXED DOLLAR AMOUNT

Obviously, it would be nice to know now what you will pay down the road if you are offered the opportunity to buy into the practice. A price based on a fixed dollar amount gives you certainty in that regard. However, a fixed dollar amount is rarely a good deal for you in the long run. It can usually be described in one of two ways. It is either a ridiculously low price or a randomly chosen number based on what the partners feel the practice is worth. A ridiculously low potential purchase price for a piece of the practice probably has lots of appeal to you now. However, a low buy-in price is probably not in your best interest.

Some practices base the buy-in price on the "par value" of the practice's stock. "Par value" is a legal/accounting term that reflects the stock's value set forth in the practice's incorporation document. Par value has no

93

significance whatsoever in determining the shares' market value. However, I occasionally encounter practices that are willing to sell you an ownership interest based on the par value of the practice's stock. You may actually end up owning a major percentage of a very lucrative practice for as little as $100. What's not to like about a deal like that? Plenty.

When a partner retires or leaves the practice, the buy-out amount for his or her shares is usually the same as the buy-in amount. As great as it is to buy-in cheaply, it really hurts to sell your shares for a pittance. This is a twofold problem. First, in the long term, when it is time for you to leave the practice you will be selling your shares for next to nothing. After you have devoted your entire career to building the practice's value, leaving with a handshake and a check for $100 hardly seems fair.

Second, there is a greater, shorter-term problem with shares that are valued at a much lower amount than their true value. As I've said before, healthcare in this country runs in cycles. At the time of this writing, the United States is experiencing a long-term cycle in which hospitals are buying private practices. Private practices are selling in droves and owners are becoming hospital-employed physicians. The selling physicians, of course, refer patients to the buying hospital before and (especially) after they sell the practice to the hospital. Accordingly, fraud and abuse laws, as we discussed in Chapter 1, require the hospital to pay fair market value for the practice.

When a hospital buys a practice, that practice's physicians naturally refer patients to the buying hospital before and after the sale. Accordingly, fraud and abuse laws require the hospital to pay fair market value for the practice.

A thorough discussion of the valuation of medical practices goes well beyond the scope of this book. However, suffice it to say that very few medical practices will be valued at an amount anywhere near their shares' par value. The practice's hard assets are likely to be worth many thousands of dollars. More importantly, medical practices, like any other business, have a component of value for "goodwill." Goodwill value in a medical practice consists of several intangible assets, including patient base, reputation, location, size, specialty, and payor mix.

Because of all the variables involved in calculating goodwill values, there aren't any hard and fast rules. However, the value of goodwill is frequently determined based on a percentage of the previous year's total revenue. If the average physician in a primary care practice is generating $1,600,000 of revenue in a year, the goodwill attributable to that physician can be expected to be approximately $400,000 if goodwill is calculated at 25% of revenue (a fair benchmark). To the extent that physicians in other specialties generate more revenue, of course, the goodwill value of their practices will increase proportionately.

As a new physician in a practice, you have to be concerned that an older physician-owner (whose buy-sell agreement in the practice might give him $100 when he leaves) will be sorely tempted to sell to a nearby hospital and receive hundreds of thousands of dollars for goodwill, plus a portion of the value of the practice's hard assets (furniture, equipment, etc.). Given the enormous spread between what the practice will eventually pay for the physician's shares and what that physician can get from the hospital immediately, many physicians in that position will choose to sell to the hospital.

It would be wrong to assume that this problem will go away when the current wave of hospital purchases dies down. Once the market decides that private practices are viable again (and, if history is any guide, this will be the next big thing), you can expect to see another rise of physician practice management companies (PPMCs).

PPMCs are publicly traded companies that "roll up" (i.e., buy and combine) multiple private practices in a given specialty. The idea behind these entities is that the purchased practices will generate more money for the owners through centralized billing, supply and equipment purchases, and management. Because PPMCs are publicly traded, they can give their own stock as partial consideration for the purchase price of the practices they are buying. The last time PPMCs were big, they were able to offer as much as 1.2 times the previous year's gross revenue for a practice[9]. Thus, the average primary care physician generating $1,600,000 of annual gross revenue might expect to receive as much as $1,920,000 for his or her shares. A physician in a specialty that generates more revenue would naturally see his or her shares valued at an even higher amount. When the difference between what a PPMC is offering immediately and what the physician would get if he or she stayed in the practice (and accepted a nominal buy-out at retirement) approaches seven figures, the PPMC offer is going to look very enticing.

I have represented lucrative practices that split apart when the partners were presented with an eye-popping offer from a PPMC. In one case, the physicians had all bought into the practice at nominal consideration (a few hundred dollars) and had a buy-sell agreement that would provide the same payment to them at retirement. When presented with an offer from the PPMC that valued each shareholder's shares at more than a million dollars, the partners split over what to do. The older physicians, who were closer to retirement, vehemently argued for selling to the PPMC; they would gain thousands of times more than what they would get from the practice under their buy-sell agreement. The younger physicians, who were doing quite well and wanted to retain their independence, strongly argued to reject the offer.

---

[9] This was the multiple used in several practice sales I was involved in during the Roaring 90s.

Ultimately, and unsurprisingly, the practice disintegrated. The younger physicians left to form a new practice and ended up competing with their former partners. Once genial colleagues became bitter enemies overnight. This horrible situation could have been avoided if they had adopted a fairer method for the valuation of their shares.

A similar problem arises when the practice picks a random dollar amount that the partners decide is the shares' "value." This number may or may not accurately reflect the true market value of shares when it is chosen. Even if it was accurate at the time, it is highly unlikely that this valuation will remain accurate through the life of the practice. If the valuation is too high, you end up paying more than your shares are worth. If the valuation is too low, you are in a situation similar to that of paying par value for your shares.

Many physicians think that agreeing to pay the shares' fair market value when they buy-in to the practice will solve the problems associated with agreeing to pay a fixed dollar amount. However, this valuation method has its own unique issues.

FAIR MARKET VALUE

At first blush, agreeing to pay the fair market value for your shares if and when you are offered partnership may seem eminently reasonable. In a perfect world, this would be the ideal price for the current owners to sell and for you to buy. Unfortunately, this isn't a perfect world. Imagine you have worked at a practice for some time, so the current owner or owners have had the opportunity to check on you for one or more years. The owners feel you are a good fit for the practice professionally, as well as a good fit for them personally. You are now offered an ownership interest.

If your initial employment agreement provided that you would pay the fair market value for your shares, it will now be up to you and the owners to figure out what that number is. There are three possible approaches that the owners could use to figure out the shares' market value.

First, the owners (who are, it should be noted, physicians, not appraisers) could just come up with a valuation on their own. Human nature being what it is, this valuation is likely to be a smidgen on the high side. You will then be faced with either accepting that offer or attempting to persuade the owners to lower it. Since you are no more qualified than they are to assign a value to a medical practice, this process may involve very heated negotiations in which tempers can flare. Receiving the offer of partnership, which should be a happy moment in your life, can then lead to a very unhappy process. Sometimes the owners and the employed physician are unable to work out their differences over the value of the shares, and the new physician either remains an employee or leaves the practice. I feel very strongly that the time to negotiate with the practice is *before* you sign your first employment agreement, when you have other options – not after you have built a patient base and are truly accepted as a colleague by the practice's other physicians.

The time to negotiate terms of ownership is *before* you sign your employment agreement, not after you have built a patient base and the other physicians have truly accepted you as a colleague.

A second method sometimes used to attempt to determine a practice's fair market value is to have the practice hire an appraiser and insist that the price you pay should be the valuation as determined by that appraiser. This also seems reasonable at first blush. The problem is that there are several widely accepted approaches to valuing a practice, and appraisers tend to select the approach that favors their client. One of the highest qualifications for a real estate appraiser is the MAI designation, and an old joke in the industry holds that this designation stands for "Made As Instructed."[10] Accordingly, you are likely to be displeased with the valuation determined by an appraiser hired by the practice, and heated negotiations can ensue.

A third approach to determining the practice's fair market value is to have both sides (you and the practice) each hire an appraiser. The price can then be determined by splitting the difference, since the "MAI phenomenon" discussed above will likely result in two widely different values. If I can't dissuade the practice from using the fair

---

[10] This is not meant to be derogatory to any particular appraiser or the industry. Most appraisers are wonderful, caring people who are working to make the world a better place.

market value method, I will usually attempt to negotiate this approach. Although splitting the difference between the two appraisers' values is unlikely to satisfy either side completely, the alternative is a heated negotiation – not a happy spot for you at this phase of your career.

Because of the almost inevitable conflicts in using the fair market value approach to determining the buy-in price, many practices use approaches that are based on the book value of the shares at the time they are offered to you.

BOOK VALUE

This is the valuation approach that I prefer. Practices that value shares based on book value can often arrive at the purchase price of shares just by sitting down with the practice manager or lead physician and looking at the balance sheet. Having two physicians sit down with calculators to arrive at the purchase price of shares is infinitely better for their future relationship than having them sit down with two lawyers, as well as possibly two accountants and two appraisers. It's also a whole lot cheaper.

You can calculate a share's book value in its purest form by subtracting the practice's liabilities from its assets and dividing that total by the number of shares. For example, if the practice had $110,000 of assets on the books (e.g., accounts receivable, furniture, and equipment) and had a line of credit outstanding of $10,000, the practice's book value would be $100,000. If the practice had 100 shares of stock outstanding, the value of each share would be $1,000.

101

Therefore, if you were going to own 25% of the practice, you would buy 25 shares at $1,000 each, with a total purchase price of $25,000. The calculation would look like this:

Book value of assets	$110,000
Less liabilities	(-10,000)
Total book value of practice	$100,000
Total number of shares outstanding	100
Total value of each share	$1,000

The book value method can result in rather high buy-in prices if the practice owns real estate or expensive medical equipment. In these cases, the book value of the real estate or medical equipment would be counted in the practice's assets. In the above example, assume the practice (in addition to the $110,000 of accounts receivable, furniture, and equipment already discussed) also owns the building it uses. The book value of this building would also be included in the assets' book value. Thus, a building valued on the books at $500,000 would bring the total book value of the practice's assets to $610,000. The practice's total book value would also be reduced by the amount of any mortgage or other indebtedness related to the property. Therefore, if the practice had a $400,000 mortgage on the building, the calculation of the book value of shares would look like this:

Book value of assets	$610,000
Less liabilities	(-410,000)
Total book value of practice	$200,000
Total number of shares outstanding	100
Total value of each share	$2,000

There are many variations. A common one is to exclude the practice's accounts receivable from the calculation of assets and to pay these accounts receivable to the current partners. The effect of this variation is to reduce the purchase price, since the book value of the assets is now less. For example, if the practice had $100,000 of accounts receivable on its books, the calculation would look like this:

Book value of assets	$610,000
Less liabilities	(-410,000)
Less accounts receivable	(-100,000)
Total book value of practice	$100,000
Total number of shares outstanding	100
Total value of each share	$1,000

Another common variation of the book value method relates to practices that keep their books on a tax basis. Many practices keep their books on a tax basis. That is, the practice's books reflect expenses that are based on tax accounting principles, rather than generally accepted accounting principles. The advantage to this method of bookkeeping is that the practice's income statement matches its tax return. Practices using the tax basis bookkeeping system sometimes make adjustments to the value of assets shown on the books for purposes of calculating the value of shares.

For example, in 2019 a business may be able to purchase up to $1,000,000 of equipment and write it off entirely (i.e., treat the entire cost of the equipment as an expense on its tax return) in the year of purchase. Therefore, an expensive piece of equipment purchased the previous year may not be carried as an asset on the books the current year, since the entire price of the equipment was treated as an expense the previous year. Generally accepted accounting principles (carefully developed over many years to reflect the most accurate method of keeping books) would not allow a write-off such as this: the treatment of an asset's purchase price as an expense is a figment of the U.S. tax system. If a practice bought an x-ray machine last year, that machine likely isn't worthless this year.

Therefore, some practices using a tax basis of accounting will adjust the practice's book value for the purpose of setting a purchase price of shares, making the balance sheet closer to what it would look like if the practice used generally accepted accounting principles. Those practices adjust the value of hard assets and treat them as declining in value equally over some number of years. Accountants call this "straight-line depreciation." For example, if a $25,000 piece of equipment were purchased the previous year and treated as an expense that year, the asset would not be reflected in the practice's book value. For the purpose of calculating the shares' purchase price, though, the practice may assume this equipment will be useful for five years, so it still has four years of value left. In this case, the practice would calculate the value of this asset for purposes of developing a share purchase price the current year as $20,000 ($25,000 x 4/5). If the other numbers were the same as those in the prior example, the calculation of the purchase price would look like this:

Book value of assets	$610,000
Less liabilities	(-410,000)
Less accounts receivable	(-100,000)
Plus value of asset expensed last year	$20,000
Total book value of practice	$120,000
Total number of shares outstanding	100
Total value of each share	$1,200

The ability to treat assets as expenses in the year of purchase is not the only incentive in the tax code designed to encourage investment. The tax code also allows accelerated depreciation, which means businesses can take a tax deduction for the cost of assets that the practice did not expense more quickly than in the straight-line depreciation used in generally accepted accounting principles. Therefore, practices that keep their books on a tax basis may also adjust the value of assets on their books for purposes of determining the purchase price for shares: they do this by adjusting the value of these assets to assume an equal decline in value over some assumed useful life (i.e., they adjust the assets' value to the value they would have if straight-line depreciation had been used).

For example, assume the practice purchased $20,000 of assets two years ago and did not expense these assets. Instead, the practice took accelerated depreciation on the assets. The calculation of those assets' value might include adding back in the accelerated depreciation taken and subtracting the straight-line depreciation that would have been taken if the practice used generally accepted accounting principles. Carrying forward the same numbers from the hypothetical practice that we have been using, the calculation of the shares' value would now look like this:

Book value of assets	$610,000
Less liabilities	(-410,000)
Less accounts receivable	(-100,000)
Plus value of asset expensed last year	20,000
Plus tax depreciation on asset purchased 2 years ago	12,200
Minus straight-line depreciation on asset purchased 2 years ago	(-4,000)
Total book value of practice	$128,200
Total number of shares outstanding	100
Total value of each share	$1,282

THE BOTTOM LINE ON BUY-INS

There are many ways that practices value their shares. Alternative methods of valuation might be preferable, but if the existing partners have executed a buy-sell agreement (and they better have!), then the practice is not likely to be inclined to change how it values shares. Whatever the valuation method for your buy-in, it is important, from your perspective, that the buy-out method (i.e., the way your shares will be valued when you retire or otherwise leave the practice) matches the buy-in method. For this reason, I always request a copy of the current buy-sell agreement among the owners when negotiating.

When I negotiate agreements with private practices, I also request a copy of the practice's financials. I have had mixed success in that regard. For most physicians accepting positions at private practices, eventual ownership is one of the biggest concerns. Since owning a piece of the pie is so crucial to my client, I feel it is reasonable to find out if it is a good pie (i.e., if the practice is financially sound). I have seen practices where the owners have maintained unrealistic salaries by drawing on a line of credit over many years. If the practice can't support reasonable salaries, you may not want to hitch your wagon to that practice. In addition, you probably don't want to become liable for debt that was incurred to inflate somebody else's salary.

However, most practices are very reluctant to share their financial information with a physician who isn't even an employee yet. Persuading practices to share such confidential information is frequently one of the biggest challenges in negotiations.

If it is your understanding that if you become a partner, you will become an equal partner, then that stipulation should be explicitly included in the agreement. In addition, you need to examine the practice's governance documents to determine whether you will have an equal vote in important matters concerning the practice. The governance documents are generally contained in the bylaws of a corporation or the operating agreement of a limited liability company (LLC).

There are nearly endless variations on how practices bring in new partners. The goal for negotiations of your employment agreement in that regard is not to get the practice to change its internal governance systems or financial practices. Instead, the goal is to ensure the following:

- There is a provision in your employment agreement that discusses your potential ownership in the practice if the stars align;
- That provision sets forth a method for the valuation of the buy-in; and
- The buy-in valuation method matches the buy-out valuation method.

Negotiations over provisions regarding your potential ownership can be some of the trickiest you will encounter. As somebody who isn't even hired yet, you may have a difficult time persuading the practice to let you peek behind the curtain and see its intimate financial details. These negotiations require diplomacy and openness from both parties.

(If a hospital is not involved in recruiting you to the private practice, so you don't have a recruitment agreement involved with your employment, please feel free to skip to the Conclusion, where we will discuss negotiation strategies.)

RECRUITMENT AGREEMENTS

Many health systems address perceived deficiencies in physician specialties in their service area by assisting private practices to recruit physicians into the area. These physician recruitment agreements can be a boon to both the

109

practice and you, and often allow a practice to be able to afford to bring in a physician it would otherwise be unable to recruit.

One common form of physician recruitment agreement constitutes an income guarantee for the practice and/or you. In simple terms, the agreement guarantees that the practice will receive enough income from your services to pay you your salary and benefits, and costs directly attributable to your practice. To the extent you do not generate collections sufficient to cover these costs, the health system agrees to pay the deficit to the practice. This is generally structured as a loan. Typically there is a "guarantee period" and a "repayment period." During the guarantee period the health system advances funds to the extent needed to pay your salary and benefits, and costs directly attributable to your practice. Generally, no payment is made by the hospital in a given month if collections are adequate to pay these costs, but no repayment of prior advances is required either. Sometimes the practice then pays back the amounts advanced by the health system in future months (the "repayment period"), but frequently the amounts paid are treated as a loan. If the hospital payments are treated as a loan, the hospital advances are ratably forgiven over the repayment period.

There is always a requirement that you stay in the geographical area for some period of time - usually the repayment period. I try to limit this requirement as much as possible. Once your income is no longer guaranteed, your employment becomes less assured by the practice. Hopefully, you will have developed your own practice by then – but if you haven't for some reason (for example, if the practice had an issue with an impaired physician that significantly reduced referrals), you could be forced to leave and thereby trigger a repayment obligation to the hospital.

There are frequently detailed provisions concerning what expenses will be allocated to you. It is important to ensure that this is a comprehensive list of expenses. For example, expenses should include: lease or rental charges for space and equipment solely utilized by you; reasonable utility and telephone expenses (including expenses of a cell phone and usage plan); malpractice insurance premiums; medical staff dues; medical and office supplies; a portion of premiums for general casualty and liability insurance; reasonable billing, collection, legal, accounting and other professional fees related to you personally; CME expenses; mileage allowances for trips between offices and hospitals; medical association dues; licensure and DEA fees; board certification and recertification costs; health, disability and life insurance premiums; and medical school debt assistance. While not every practice will provide each of those benefits, I try to get these benefits inserted into the recruitment agreement (and your employment agreement) while the practice is using "other people's money."

Although all monies are usually paid to the practice, the health system usually treats you as a co-borrower. Frequently you can limit the circumstances under which you personally would be required to repay advances. However, it is difficult to argue that you should not be responsible for repayment of the loan where you have terminated your employment agreement without cause.

The health system generally protects its investment in several ways. First, it will take a security interest on the accounts receivable of the practice. Provisions regarding the security interest must be carefully analyzed. Many times the health system will attempt to insert a security interest on **all** accounts receivable of the practice. This can frequently be negotiated to only cover the accounts receivable generated by you.

The health system will usually also require repayment of amounts advanced if your employment is terminated for any reason. Two considerations apply here. First, repayment should generally come from the practice, not you. The practice received the income guarantee so that it could pay you a reasonable salary for services rendered. The expectation of any private practice is that ultimately it will profit from the services of its employed physicians. I have been able to negotiate a clause to the effect that any repayment will come solely from accounts receivable generated by the physician, unless the employment agreement is terminated without cause by the physician. The second consideration only applies to the extent you are unable to negotiate total personal relief from repayment obligations. At a minimum in these circumstances you should be relieved from repayment if your employment agreement is terminated because of your death or disability.

As is the case with sign-on bonuses, there are tax consequences to receipt of these payments from the hospital. Since the payments are structured as a loan when they are received, they are not taxable income to you or the practice as received. However, as the loans are forgiven, the amount forgiven is treated as taxable income. It is my opinion that since the payment was made to the practice to allow it to hire a revenue-generator (you), the taxable income generated from loan forgiveness should be attributed to the practice.

Conclusion: The Wisdom of Experience

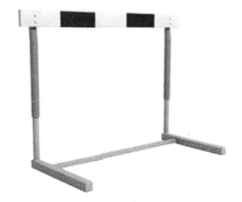

Conclusion

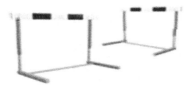

Accepting your first medical position is a milestone in your life. It is the culmination of all the efforts you have put forth since high school to earn the title of "Doctor." You should be very proud of yourself.

To enhance your well-earned satisfaction, you want to make sure that your new employment relationship is fair for both you and the employer. I hope this book will assist you in obtaining a position that meets both your personal and professional needs.

Let's sum up the high points and talk about where you need to go from here.

As I discussed in Chapter 1, it is extremely important that you obtain an objective compensation analysis in order to ascertain that the compensation offered is in line with that offered to other similarly situated physicians (those in your specialty, in the area). I also discussed the crucial relationship between the compensation offered and the amount of work the employer will expect from you to earn that compensation. The employer offering the biggest compensation package probably expects the most work from you. Balancing your lifestyle choices with the employer's needs may be impossible if you accept a position from an employer that expects peak productivity.

You are now familiar with the ugly downsides that accompany productivity-based compensation in the early years of employment and with the various types of productivity formulas frequently used by employers. Once again, I urge you not to accept pure productivity-based compensation in the first year of your employment if there are other options available.

When evaluating a compensation package, never assume that you will qualify for bonus compensation. Don't be seduced into a position with "adequate" compensation by rationalizing that your bonus will make it acceptable.

I discussed what benefits you may expect to receive in addition to your compensation and how to compare benefits offered by different employers. I also talked about the balancing act between the employer's need to retain flexibility over benefits provided by a third party (e.g., health insurance and disability insurance) and your need to avoid the employer's unilateral amendment of important benefits (e.g., vacation). The requirements of tax law concerning qualified retirement plans generally prevent employers from negotiating provisions relating to those plans.

A frequent trap for both employers and employees who are not represented by an experienced physicians' contract attorney involves payments that are in some way directly or indirectly tied to the value or volume of referrals from the physician to the employer. Since fraud and abuse laws make it illegal to pay or accept payment for referrals of federal health programs' beneficiaries, you need to be alert to any potential violations of these laws.

In Chapter 2 I discussed the devastating impact that restrictive covenants can have on your career. Given the healthcare environment's volatility, you should never assume that the first position you accept will end up being the workplace where you will spend your entire career. A restrictive covenant may force you to leave an established patient base after a few years and start your career over in a new area. Having to move to a new area can have a major impact on your personal life (and your family's lives) as well as your professional life. Before you agree to anything, you need to make sure that you can still earn a living in your location if things don't work out with your first employer.

The restrictive covenant should only prohibit locating your new office in the restricted area; it should not prohibit the practice of medicine in that area. In other words, you should be able to see patients in a hospital that is in the restricted area, as long as your office is not in the restricted area. A reasonable restriction would prohibit opening an office within a radius of five miles from any location where you spent a significant amount of your time while employed by your former employer. A one-year restriction is common, but sometimes you can negotiate a provision that the restriction should last either the amount of time you worked for the employer or one year, whichever is less. The geographical area may be larger for subspecialists and for physicians practicing in a rural area.

In general, you should not agree to give up facility privileges if you leave employment. However, giving up hospital privileges may be required if you are working for a practice that has an exclusive agreement with that hospital. You may also have to give up privileges at a facility owned by a private practice that has a closed staff (in other words, a place where only that practice's physicians have privileges).

Sometimes you can buy out of a restrictive covenant. If so, try to obtain an agreement that provides that the buy-out cost decreases over time. In the first year or so, you will be leaving with patients that really belong to the employer, but over time you will develop your own patient base. Accordingly, it is reasonable to pay more to buy out a restrictive covenant in the early part of your employment, while arguably less reasonable to pay a high price after you have developed your own patient base.

Never assume that a restrictive covenant is so unreasonable that it will not be enforced if it goes to trial.

Although you may very well be right, a potential future employer is likely to want to avoid the prospect that your former employer could sue both you and your new employer. You're likely to be passed over for some other physician who doesn't come with such legal baggage.

As I discussed in Chapter 3, the purpose of a written employment agreement is to remove any doubts about what is expected of both you and the employer. The agreement should provide the patient contact hours that will be expected of you and how call coverage will be allocated. Larger employers may be able to be fairly specific in this regard, but smaller employers will probably need to retain significantly more flexibility in determining both patient contact hours and call coverage. In either case, the employer should agree to allocate call coverage equitably among all qualified providers.

Your agreement will almost certainly provide that you will not be able to start employment until you are licensed in the applicable state. The agreement may also require you to obtain privileges at one or more facilities and to be credentialed by major third-party payors as a condition of starting employment. Be mindful of the fact that credentialing conducted by facilities and (to a lesser extent) by managed care plans can move at a snail's pace. Ideally, your agreement will allow some wiggle room for negotiations if you don't have privileges at all the required facilities or aren't credentialed by all the required third-party payors at the intended start date.

I discussed the difference between for cause and not for cause terminations of employment. The delineation of grounds justifying for cause termination by the employer is one of the most crucial aspects of your agreement. Ideally, the employer will not be able to terminate your employment merely because you are accused (as opposed to being convicted) of a crime. Similarly, it is more reasonable to agree that you may be terminated if your hospital or other facility privileges are revoked, rather than if you are merely in a due process proceeding that is reviewing hospital privileges.

The definition of "disability" and the method for determining whether you are considered "disabled" are also both highly important. The employer should not be able to unilaterally determine that you are disabled, nor should the employer be permitted to choose a physician to make this determination without your concurrence.

The agreement may provide that a party has an opportunity to "cure" an alleged breach of the agreement before the other party may terminate the agreement for cause. However, some things (such as convictions or termination of hospital privileges) will generally not be treated as "curable."

Both you and the employer will generally want the ability to terminate the agreement without cause (although if you are in the United States on a J-1 visa, termination of employment might require you to leave the country, so without cause termination provisions would not be appropriate for you). You and the employer should be given the same rights regarding without cause termination. In particular, each of you should be required to give the same amount of advance notice of without cause termination. Although 90 days' notice of without cause termination is common, you should attempt to get a longer notice period if possible. You will be hard-pressed to obtain suitable replacement employment without a gap in earnings if you only have 90 days to obtain a new position.

In Chapter 4 I discussed the difference between occurrence and claims-made malpractice insurance and the importance of obtaining a provision in your employment agreement relating to payment for tail coverage (coverage for claims that are made after a claims-made policy ends) when your employment agreement terminates. Tail coverage can cost as much as a third of a year's salary. If the agreement is silent about who pays for the tail, you could end up having to pay for it. If so, you could be stuck in a job you hate, just because you can't afford to leave and pay for the tail. If the employer will not agree to pay the entire tail coverage premium, you may be able to persuade the employer to pay some portion of the tail coverage premium for every year you work there. For example, if the employer agrees to pay a fifth of the tail coverage premium for every year of service, you won't have to pay anything for the tail if you stick around for five years.

In Chapter 5 I discussed the wonderful world of private practice. The biggest difference between an employment agreement with a private practice and an employment agreement with any other employer is the potential that you could eventually become an owner of the private practice. It isn't realistic to expect to be guaranteed ownership, but your first employment agreement should have specific provisions about when you will be considered for partnership and how the buy-in's purchase price will be calculated if you are offered partnership. There aren't any discernible patterns in the variations among practices concerning the time the practice will make you wait until you are offered partnership. The time you will have to wait will most likely be based on how long the founder made the first employed physician wait.

Although there are countless variations of the methods for calculating the purchase price of a practice buy-in, these methods can generally be broken down into three classifications: payment of a fixed dollar amount, payment of fair market value, and payment of book value.

A fixed dollar amount (especially a low one) may seem appealing to you now, but there are many downsides. The buy-out price for the current owners, when they leave the practice, is usually calculated the same way as the buy-in price for new physicians. If the buy-out price for departing physicians is considerably less than what the practice is really worth, there is a risk that a hospital may offer to buy the practice and pay the current owners the practice's fair market value. In the case of a publicly traded physician practice management company (PPMC) that is able to issue its own shares as partial consideration for the purchase price, the amount of stock and cash offered to the current owners could be quite high. If the current owners are offered considerably more than they would get if they stuck around and retired from the practice, they may sell it before you are offered partnership.

Moreover, the practice owners may have calculated a fixed dollar amount that has little or no basis in market reality. The figure quoted may or may not be what your share of the partnership would be worth when you are permitted to buy in. It is extremely unlikely that a fixed dollar amount quoted during initial employment negotiations will accurately reflect what your share of the partnership will be worth in the future, when you are actually offered partnership.

Agreeing to pay fair market value for your share of the practice is a recipe for bitter negotiations when you are offered partnership. There are several methods of valuing a medical practice, and an appraiser is likely to choose the one that results in the best price for his or her client (i.e., an appraiser hired by the practice is likely to calculate a higher value for the practice than one hired by you). If the practice insists on using fair market value to value your buy-in, you may want to propose splitting the difference between the value calculated by an appraiser hired by you and an appraiser hired by the practice.

Agreeing to pay the book value is probably the best method of determining the potential future purchase price. A pure book value calculation is simple – you subtract the practice's liabilities from the value of the assets shown on the books to arrive at the entire practice's value. You then multiply your ownership percentage times the value of the total practice to determine your buy-in price.

There are many adjustments that may be made to the pure book value in determining a buy-in price. For example, many practices remove accounts receivable from the calculation and pay the accounts receivable as of the date of the buy-in to the existing partners. In addition, many practices keep their books on a tax basis. The tax laws attempt to encourage businesses to invest in the purchase of assets by allowing these assets to be written off faster for tax purposes than generally accepted accounting principles would dictate. The effect of this accelerated depreciation is to reduce the assets' book value. Therefore, practices that keep their books on a tax basis may want to adjust the value of assets shown on the books to reflect economic reality more accurately when calculating a potential purchase price.

If you have received a recruitment agreement from a hospital, you want to limit the amount of time you are required to remain in the area after the guaranteed income period expires. A recruitment agreement may allow you greater flexibility in negotiating salary and benefits, since it will be "other people's money" the practice is dealing with (at least during the period of the income guarantee). You will also want to try to limit the security given for the loans to the accounts receivable you generate from the practice. Finally, you will want the taxable income generated from loan forgiveness to be an obligation of the practice, not you.

NOW WHAT?

You now know a lot about the most important aspects of a physician employment agreement. You probably already know that your first employment agreement is likely to have the biggest influence on your career (and life) of any contract you will ever be involved in. After all you have accomplished to get to this point in your life, it is only natural for you to expect a contract that is perfect for you. Unfortunately, the world doesn't work like that.

Although the first draft agreement that is presented to you will not be carved in stone (even though the recruiter may imply that it is), you have to recognize that the employer, just like you, has interests to protect. No matter how hard the agreement may be negotiated, it will never be perfect from your perspective. Most employers will address reasonable objections to provisions in the early drafts and will make compromises. You need to be willing to compromise as well.

Even though you can't expect a perfect contract, you must constantly bear in mind that now is the time to negotiate the terms of your employment – before you accept that employment. No matter how desperately you may want a position, you do have some leverage in negotiations before the agreement is executed. This leverage will evaporate the moment you sign on the dotted line. The people you will be negotiating with could be your colleagues soon, so tact is

127

obviously required to ensure that relationships do not become strained. Nevertheless, if you do not stand up for your rights now, you could end up paying for deficiencies in the agreement for the rest of your career.

 No matter how much you want a position, you have leverage during negotiations. This leverage ends the moment you sign on the dotted line.

Most physicians do not get the best deal possible when they are negotiating for themselves. Faced with massive debt, they naturally tend to focus entirely on monetary provisions. In effect, they mortgage their future (e.g., they agree to onerous restrictive covenants, ignore issues concerning payment for tail coverage, and so forth) in return for what strikes them as a massive paycheck immediately.

If you work too hard to avoid appearing overly aggressive during negotiations, the employer may get the impression that the issues under discussion are not really important to you. Not surprisingly, in those circumstances the employer will be unwilling to compromise significantly over these provisions. Nor should you try to impress your future colleagues by demonstrating quick decision-making in the area of contract negotiation (as you have been trained to do when making medical decisions). In contrast, experienced negotiators of physician employment agreements almost never make on-the-spot decisions – especially when reacting to a written offer prepared by the other side's attorney.

For these reasons, it is always advisable to hire an experienced physicians' contract attorney to review and potentially negotiate your contract for you. A good physicians' contract attorney will have experience that you simply don't have. There is wisdom in experience. Just as you have gained medical insights and knowledge beyond what you learned in school, an experienced physicians' contract attorney has gained insights and knowledge in practicing physician contract law.

You must retain the right attorney for this important negotiation. Contract law is a complicated area and many attorneys only dabble in it. Fraud and abuse laws, and other legal restraints on the practice of medicine, are complex and constantly changing. Assuring compliance with these laws, regulations, and interpretations of the relevant regulatory agencies adds a layer of complexity to the negotiations.

This is not a job for a generalist. You get what you pay for, and you really need an attorney who focuses on physician contract law. An experienced attorney will have been involved in win-win negotiations of physician employment agreements for many years, and during that time the attorney becomes adept at determining which variations work for both parties. Every contract an experienced attorney works on is therefore even better than the one before.

By using an experienced physicians' contract attorney to handle these delicate negotiations, you also preserve your personal relationships with your future colleagues. The beauty of using a lawyer is that you are no longer the one making the requests for changes to the agreement. If questioned about issues, you can always just blame your lawyer ("He said I shouldn't agree to this…" or "She said it should be worded this way…"). If all else fails, use the "dumb doc" approach: "I don't really understand all this legal mumbo-jumbo, so I have to rely on my attorney to work through this agreement."

There's a story about a physician who is traveling on a train. He slips off his shoes to get more comfortable on the long trip and discovers that the folks seated on his right and left are both lawyers.

After a time, the physician decides to get up and get something to drink in the café car. He asks the lawyer sitting by the aisle if he'd like anything. The lawyer says he'd love a Coke. While the physician is gone, the lawyer picks up one of the physician's shoes and spits in it.

The physician comes back and hands the lawyer his drink, and the lawyer on his other side then asks if he also could have a Coke. The physician doesn't want to be rude, so he goes to get that lawyer a drink, too. While he is off on this mission, the second lawyer picks up the physician's other shoe and spits in it.

The physician comes back, and they all make small talk until the train pulls into the station. The doctor then slips into his shoes and instantly knows what has happened.

"When will the antagonism end between our professions?" he says in exasperation. "The spitting in the shoes, the urinating in the Cokes – when will it end?"

I hope your experience with the legal profession will be somewhat kinder than that. You have come a long, long way and obtaining a reasonable employment agreement should be the final hurdle on your way to a long and prosperous career in medicine.

With luck, our paths may cross some day. If they do, I'd be honored if you'd buy me a Coke.

THE PHYSICIAN PROSPERITY PROGRAM®

A SPECIAL OFFER FOR READERS OF THIS BOOK

www.PaHealthLaw.com

You have read this book and you have a contract, what should you do now? You badly need both practical advice and expert guidance as you deal with the process of obtaining your first position. *Analyzing compensation structures and contractual terms for physician employment agreements is another "specialty" altogether, and you need a consult – stat!*

Our proprietary contract review system will give you everything you need to maximize compensation and benefits, consistent with the lifestyle you are trying to achieve.

The Contract Review System includes:

❖ Detailed compensation analysis, so you can sleep well at night, knowing you are being paid fairly, and knowing what the employer wants from you.

❖ Thorough review of the contract language by a world class physicians' contract attorney, so you know exactly what's expected of you.

❖ Professional negotiation (available as an additional service)

A WORLD CLASS PHYSICIANS' ATTORNEY WILL LOOK FOR THE HIDDEN PITFALLS THAT CAN TRAP YOU IN A BAD SITUATION

Don't let the huge dollar amount of the salary entice you to make a snap decision. We have assembled nationally recognized benchmarks to compare the salary and benefits offered against what other physicians earn in the same specialty in the same area.

The physician employment agreement you receive is not written in stone. An experienced physicians' contract attorney will give you a detailed analysis with a section-by-section breakdown of potential issues and suggested language needed for your protection, so you really understand the critical issues:

- ✓ COMPENSATION AND BENEFITS – ensure the figures are comparable to what other physicians in your specialty are getting in the area
- ✓ RESTRICTIVE COVENANTS – don't be forced to start over if things don't work out at this employer
- ✓ CALL COVERAGE – only your fair share
- ✓ DEFINING WHAT IS EXPECTED OF YOU – what kind of lifestyle will you lead?
- ✓ THE TERM OF THE AGREEMENT – are you sure you know when you start; can you get out if you don't like the employer, the situation, or other people at the employer?

- ✓ MALPRACTICE INSURANCE – will the cost of protection after you leave force you to stay in a position you hate?
- ✓ PRIVATE PRACTICE ISSUES – obtain clarity about potential future ownership.

HAVE A WORLD CLASS PHYSICIANS' ATTORNEY NEGOTIATE THE BEST DEAL – WITHOUT ALIENATING YOUR FUTURE COLLEAGUES

Additionally, if you desire it, the seasoned physician contract attorney working for you will then handle the delicate negotiations to get you the best possible deal, so you don't have to get into an adversarial relationship with your future colleagues. Physician Prosperity Program® attorneys are experienced negotiators who understand the need to maintain excellent relationships. Rest assured that the attorney will not make things awkward for you while optimizing your new employment offer.

Get a free copy of a checklist that encapsulates what you've learned in this book at www.PaHealthLaw.com/checklist

GO NOW TO SEE WHAT MOST PHYSICIANS MISS IN THEIR FIRST EMPLOYMENT AGREEMENT

www.PaHealthLaw.com

Ten Key Questions

VITAL ISSUES IN A PHYSICIAN'S EMPLOYMENT AGREEMENT

1   Is there a guaranteed salary for the first few years?
2. How many patient contact hours are expected of me each week?
3. Is there an opportunity for me to earn a bonus?
4. Besides my pay, what other benefits are available?
5. Does the agreement have a restrictive covenant in it?
6. What happens if the hospitals or managed care companies are slow to credential me?
7. How much notice will I get of without cause termination?
8. How will the employer determine disability?
9. What policies and procedures will I be required to comply with?
10. Will the employer pay all or a portion of the cost of tail coverage?

(PRIVATE PRACTICE ONLY)

a. How many years before I am considered for ownership?
b. How will my buy-in be determined?
c. If I become a partner, will I be an equal partner?

ACKNOWLEDGMENTS

This book could not have been written were it not for the hundreds of physicians who trusted me to handle one of the biggest deals of their life – their employment agreements.

Thank you to the following people:

My son, John, who, when asked to proofread the manuscript of the second edition, took it upon himself to assume the role of editor. I was shocked and delighted at the many improvements he suggested for the book.

My wife, Yvonne, who did her usual thorough job of performing a final proofreading of the manuscript.

My daughter, Rachel, for teaching me how precious life can be.

All my kids, Rachel, John, Lydia and Ben – being your Dad was the best thing that ever happened to me.

My parents, Clair and Grace Hursh, for making me who I am.

Pam Peckman, for patiently reworking the cover until it was "just right."

Made in the USA
Monee, IL
22 September 2023

43156434R00090